RICE DIET
HANDBOOK FOR WEIGHT LOSS

A Complete Guide and Solution on How to Lose Weight with Rice Diet. Including Food Lists, Recipes and a 21-Day Meal Plan.

HILDA M. JACOBS

Disclaimer:
The information provided in this book, is intended for educational purposes only. It is not a substitute for professional medical advice, diagnosis, or treatment. Always seek the advice of your physician or other qualified healthcare provider with any questions you may have regarding a medical condition.
The author and publisher of this book have made every effort to ensure that the information provided is accurate and up-to-date at the time of publication. However, medical knowledge and research are constantly evolving, and information may become outdated or subject to change. Therefore, the author and publisher do not warrant or guarantee the accuracy, completeness, or timeliness of the information presented in this book.
The author and publisher shall not be liable for any direct or indirect damages or injuries arising out of the use, interpretation, or application of any information provided in this book. Readers are encouraged to consult with their healthcare providers for individualized advice and recommendations based on their specific medical conditions and needs.

By reading this book, you acknowledge and agree to the terms of this disclaimer.
Printed in the United States of America.

First Edition: February 2024

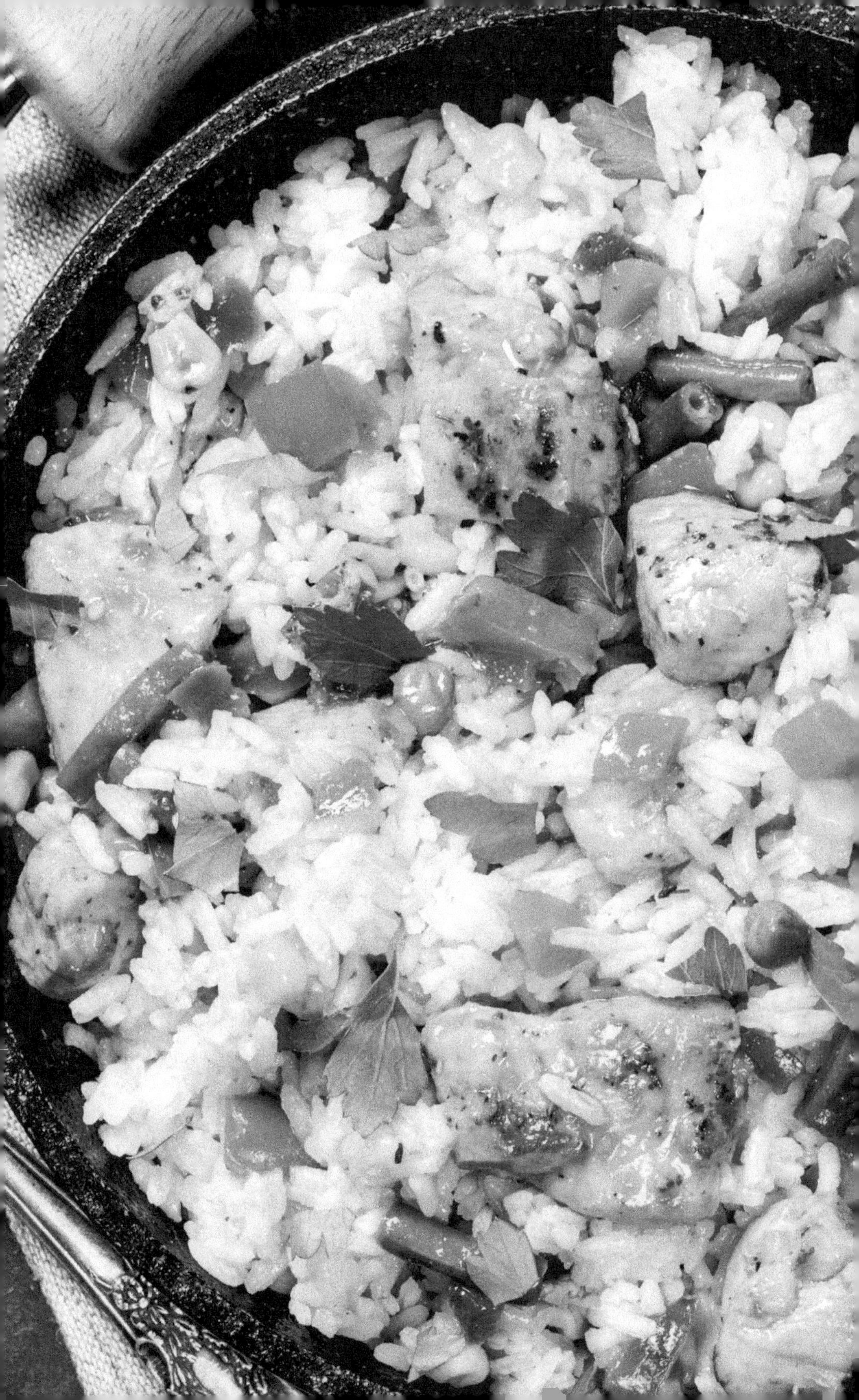

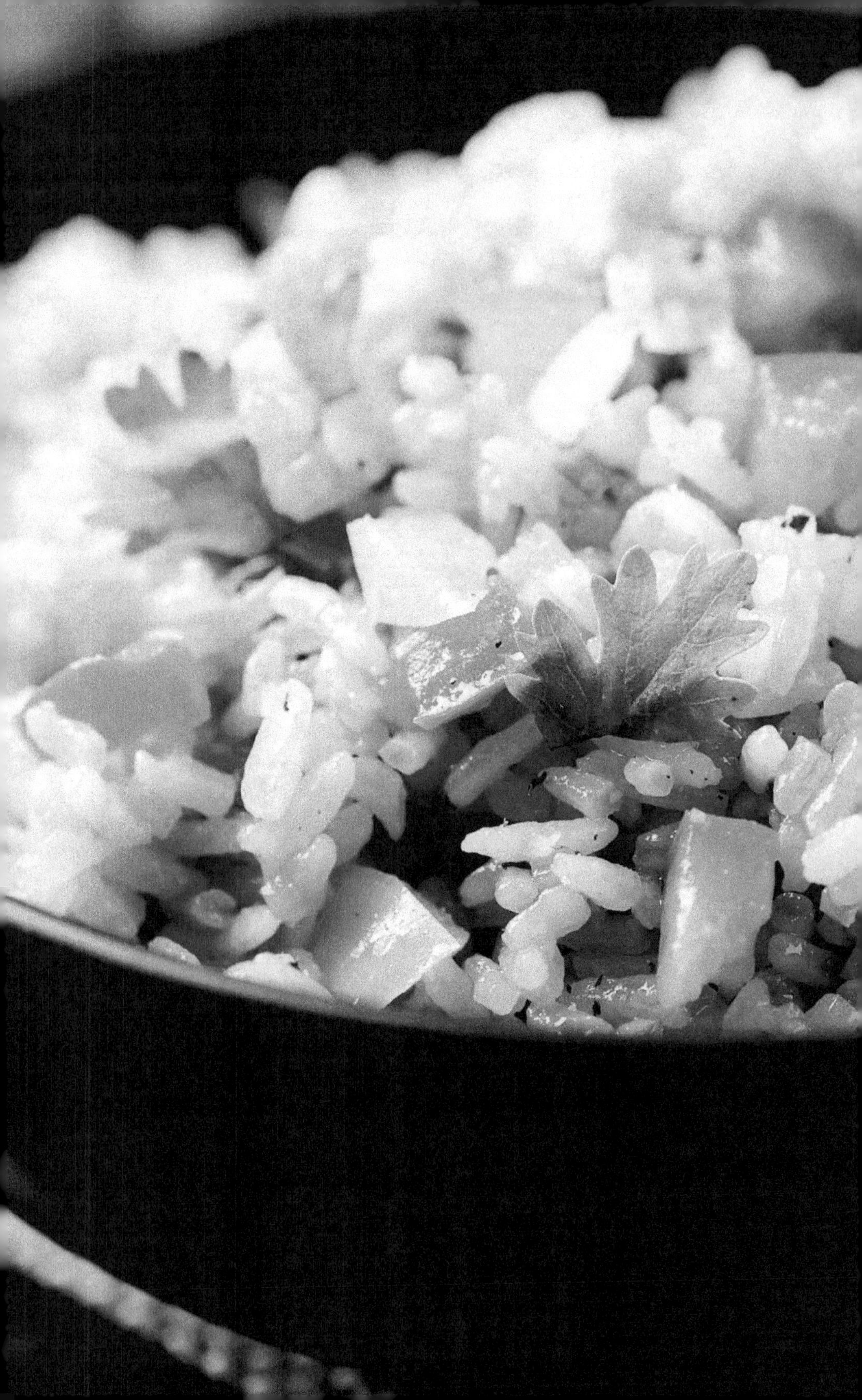

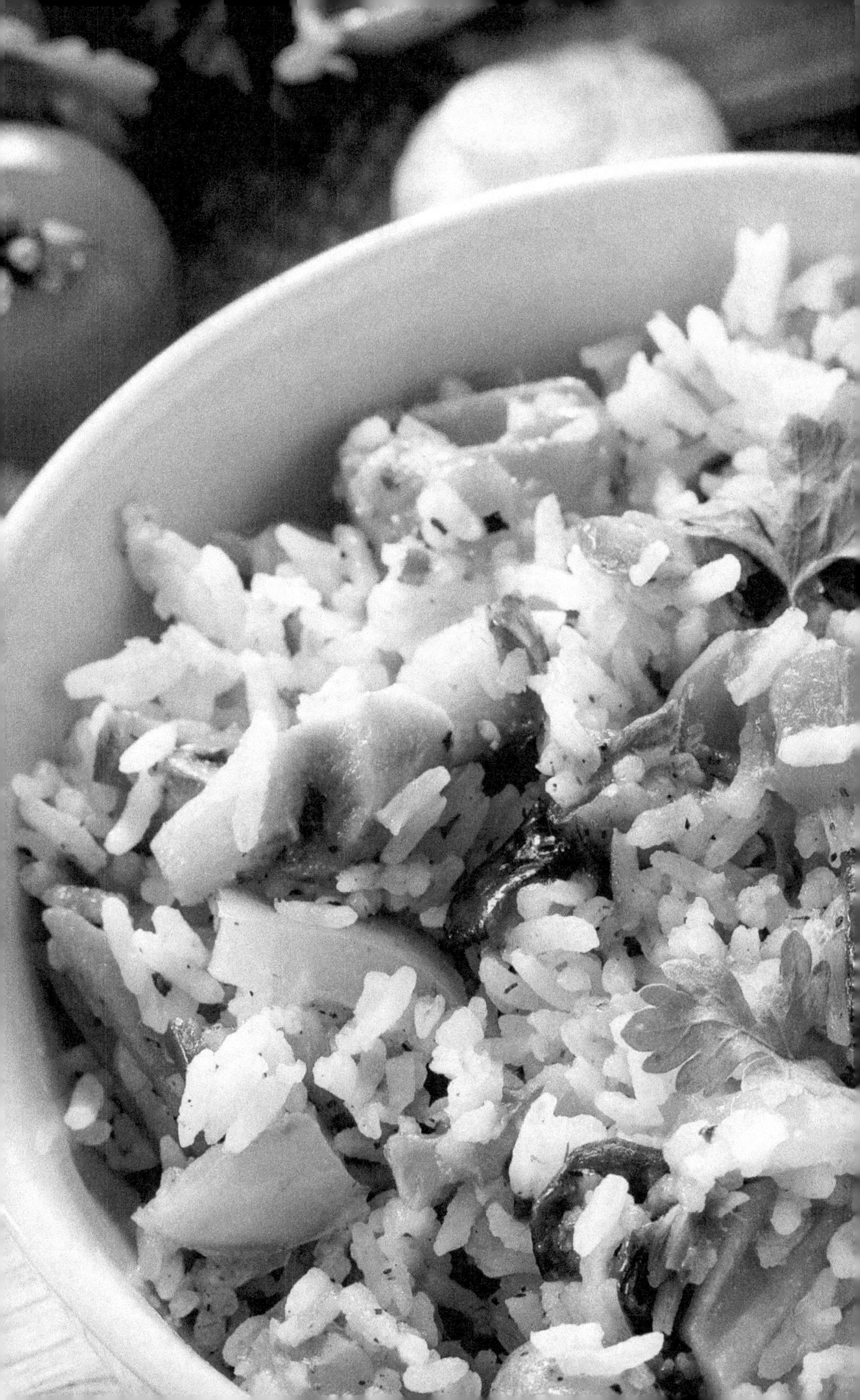

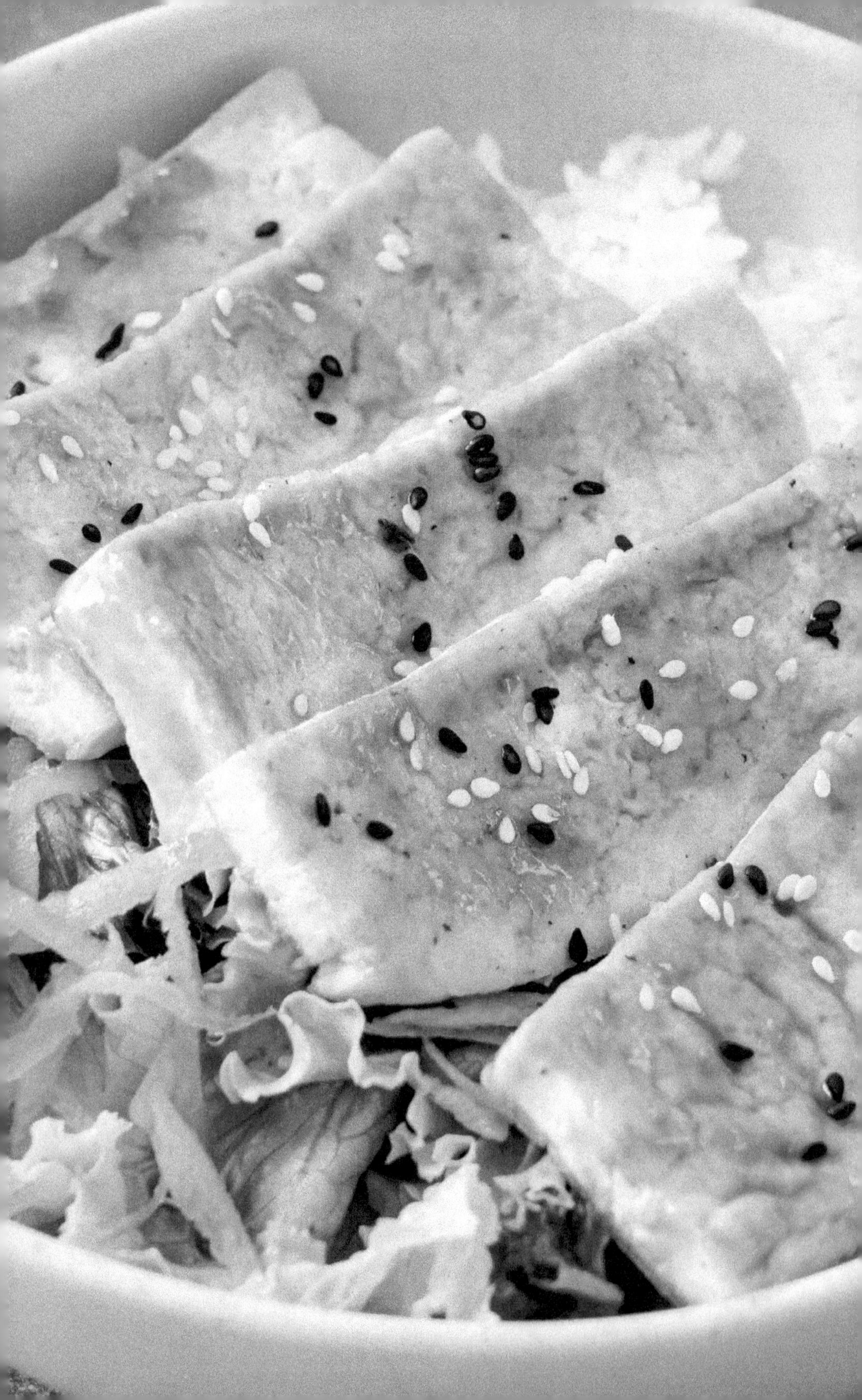

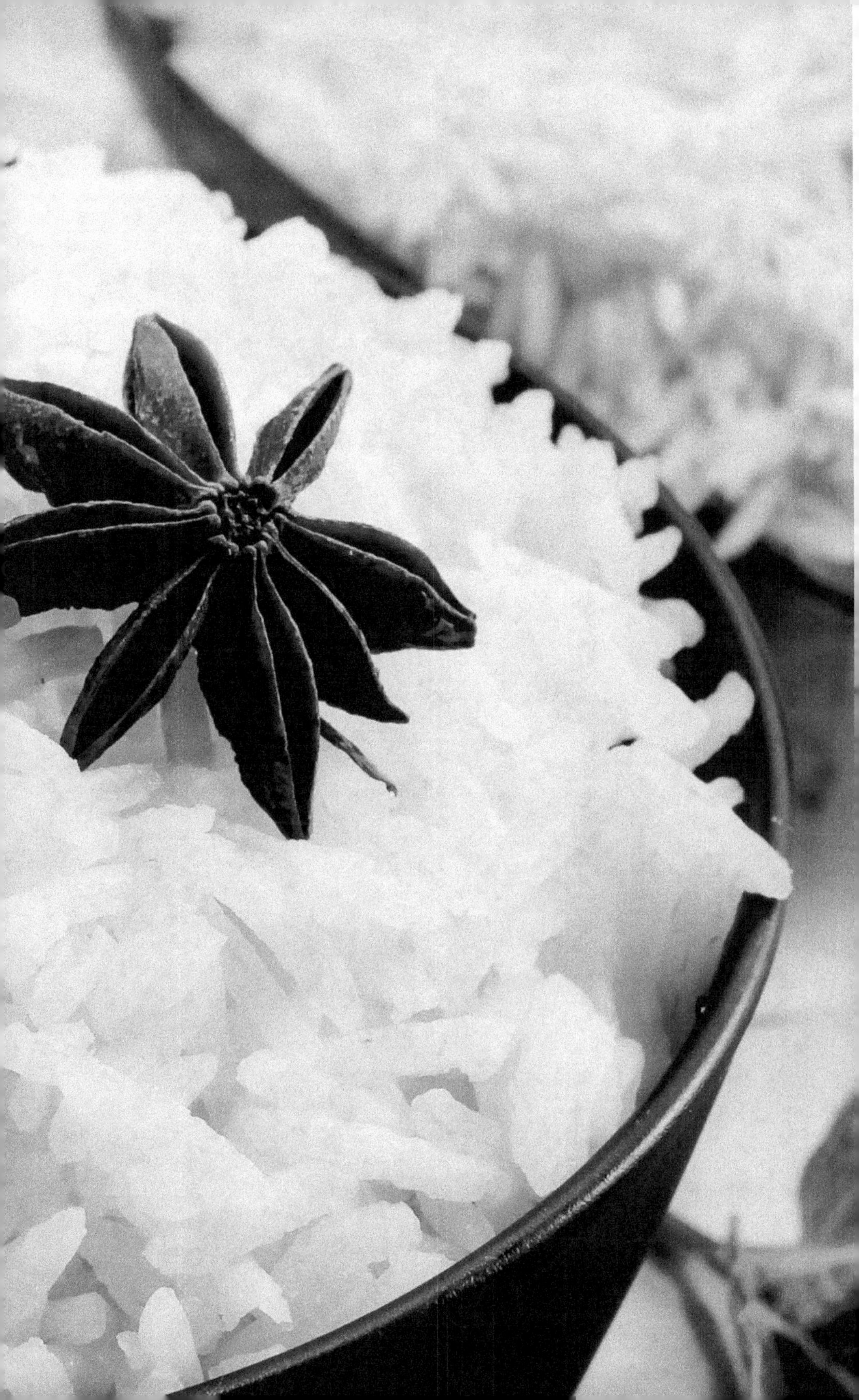

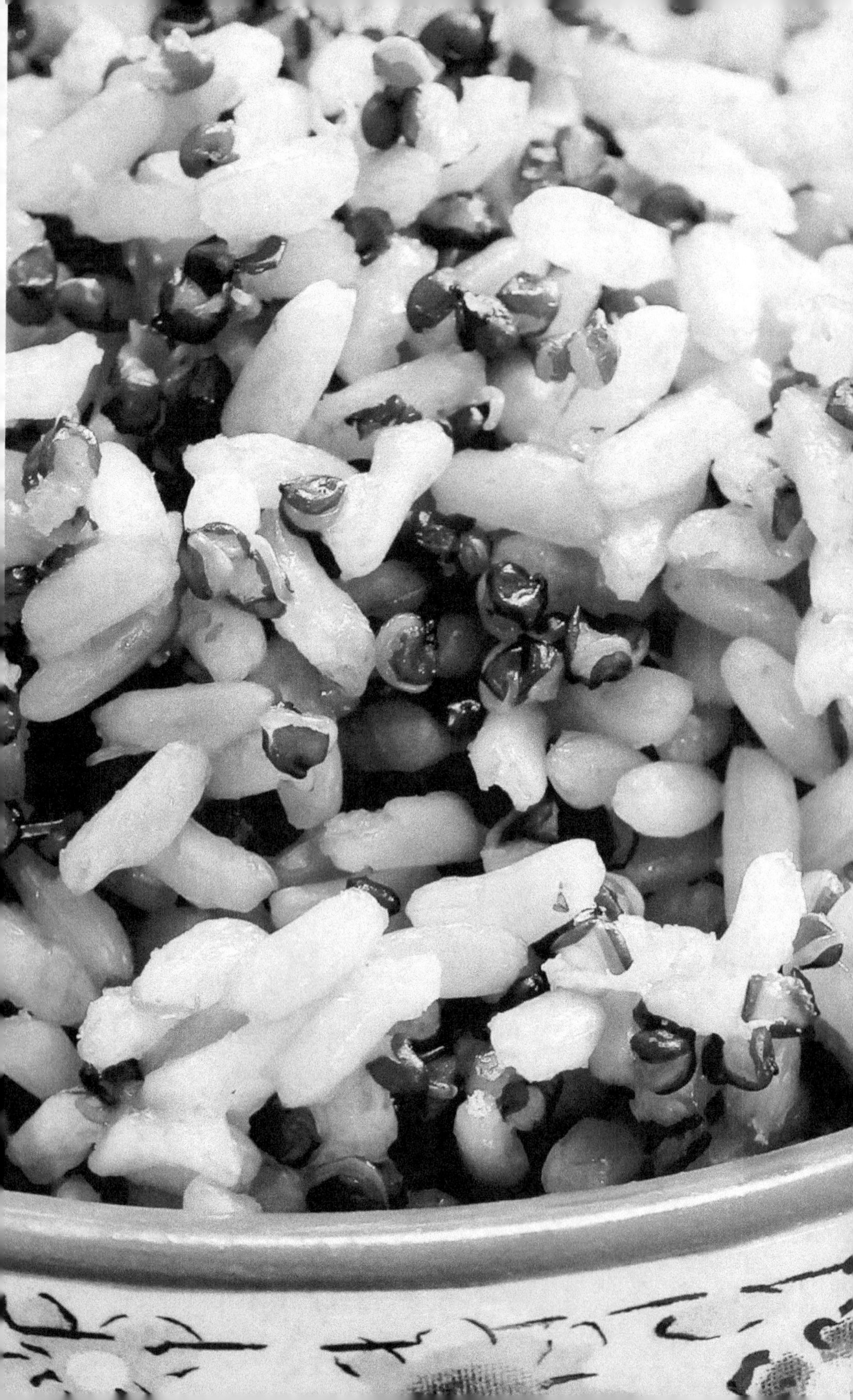

CONTENTS

INTRODUCTION..1

Overview of the Rice Diet...4

Historical Background 6

Purpose and Goals..8

THE SCIENCE BEHIND THE RICE DIET 12

Nutritional Foundations of the Rice Diet.......................12

Health Benefits..15

Weight Loss and Metabolic Improvements 22

Practical Tips for Maximizing Weight Loss and Metabolic
Benefits 24

Impact on Diabetes and Heart Disease...........................25

Implementing the Rice Diet for Diabetes and Heart Disease
Managements 27

Comparative Analysis with Other Diets 28

FOODS TO INCLUDE CHARTS IN THE RICE DIET 31

Rice Varieties 31

Fruits and Vegetables..35

Additional Plant-Based Foods 39

FOODS TO AVOID CHARTS IN THE RICE DIET 42

High-Sodium Foods 42

Fatty Foods...45

Processed and Refined Foods 47

PHASES OF THE RICE DIET 50

Phase 1 50

Phase 2 52

Phase 3 54

IMPLEMENTING THE RICE DIET 58

    Planning and Preparing Meals 58

    Managing Hunger and Cravings 60

    Dining Out and Social Events 63

    Adjustments for Personal Preferences and Nutritional Needs 66

BREAKFAST RECIPES 69

    Basic Brown Rice Porridge 69

    Fruit Salad with Lemon Mint Dressing 70

    Rice Cakes with Avocado 71

    Apple Cinnamon Rice Breakfast 72

    Tropical Rice Smoothie 73

    Peachy Rice Breakfast Bowl 74

    Savory Rice and Spinach Pancakes 75

    Rice and Berry Parfait 76

    Rice and Nutmeg Porridge 77

    Tropical Rice Pudding 78

LUNCH RECIPES 80

    Rice and Bean Salad 80

    Vegetable Stir-Fry over Brown Rice 81

    Mushroom Rice Soup 82

    Rice-Stuffed Bell Peppers 83

    Curried Rice Salad 85

    Rice and Lentil Salad 86

    Asian Rice and Cabbage Salad 87

    Mediterranean Rice Tabbouleh 88

    Rice and Chickpea Stuffed Avocados 89

    Cold Rice and Pea Soup 90

DINNER RECIPES..**92**

Lentil and Rice Stew 92

Rice Primavera...93

Cauliflower Rice Stir-Fry.......................................95

Tomato Basil Rice...96

Spinach and Lemon Rice 97

Rice and Lentil Salad 98

Asian Rice and Cabbage Salad 99

Mediterranean Rice Tabbouleh............................101

Rice and Chickpea Stuffed Avocados..................102

Cold Rice and Pea Soup.......................................103

SNACKS AND SIDES **105**

Asian Rice and Cabbage Salad 105

Mediterranean Rice Tabbouleh............................106

Rice and Chickpea Stuffed Avocados..................107

Cold Rice and Pea Soup.......................................108

Cucumber Rice Vinegar Salad 110

Rice and Zucchini Fritters....................................111

Sweet Potato Rice Cakes......................................112

Baked Rice Chips..113

Rice and Kale Chips..114

Rice and Lentil Salad 115

DESSERTS RECIPES......................................**118**

Fruit and Rice Pudding 118

Baked Apples with Rice and Cinnamon 119

Rice and Carrot Halwa 120

Rice Flour Pancakes..122

Banana Rice Cream 123

Rice and Lentil Salad 124

Asian Rice and Cabbage Salad 125

Mediterranean Rice Tabbouleh 127

Rice and Chickpea Stuffed Avocados 128

Cold Rice and Pea Soup 130

BEVERAGES RECIPES **132**

Rice Milk Smoothie 132

Golden Rice Tea 133

Rice Water with Lemon and Mint 134

Cucumber Rice Water 135

Herbal Rice Tea 137

Rice and Lentil Salad 138

Asian Rice and Cabbage Salad 139

Mediterranean Rice Tabbouleh 141

Rice and Chickpea Stuffed Avocados 142

Cold Rice and Pea Soup 143

21-DAY MEAL PLAN **145**

FREQUENTLY ASKED QUESTIONS (FAQs) **151**

Addressing Common Concerns and Misconceptions 151

CONCLUSIONS **154**

The Future of the Rice Diet 154

INTRODUCTION

Welcome to the "Rice Diet Handbook for Beginners," a journey towards a healthier, more balanced you. If you're holding this book, chances are you're looking for a change. Perhaps you've tried myriad diets, each promising the moon, yet here you are, searching still. You're not alone. The quest for a sustainable, healthful lifestyle is a road many of us walk, often with more questions than answers. That's where the Rice Diet comes in, and this handbook is your first step towards understanding and implementing a diet that's as nurturing as it is nourishing.

The Rice Diet isn't a new fad. In fact, its roots stretch back to the 1930s, a testament to its efficacy and enduring relevance. Originally developed by Dr. Walter Kempner at Duke University, the Rice Diet was a groundbreaking approach to treating chronic conditions such as hypertension, diabetes, and heart disease. Fast forward to today, and its principles remain a beacon for those seeking to reset their health compass.

At its core, the Rice Diet is simplicity itself: high in fiber, low in sodium, and rich in nutrients, all while being centered around rice, fruits, vegetables, and beans. It sounds almost too simple, doesn't it? Yet, within this simplicity lies its power. This diet isn't just about weight loss—though many have found success in shedding unwanted pounds—it's about fostering a profound, holistic change in how we approach eating and wellness.

The purpose and goals of the Rice Diet are manifold. For some, it's about managing blood pressure without the crutch of medication. For others, it's about improving kidney health, tackling diabetes, or simply seeking a lifestyle that promotes longevity and vitality. Whatever your reasons, this handbook is designed to guide you through each step, from understanding the nutritional foundations to implementing the diet in a way that fits seamlessly into your life.

Embarking on the Rice Diet is to embrace a history of wellness, drawing on decades of research and countless success stories. It's a commitment to eating whole, unprocessed foods that nourish the body and soul. But let's be clear: this isn't a magic bullet. It's a lifestyle choice, one that requires mindfulness and dedication. The good news? You don't have to do it alone. This handbook is your companion, designed to demystify the science, offer practical advice, and inspire with delicious meal ideas.

Our journey through the Rice Diet will cover its scientific underpinnings—how and why it works. We'll explore the health benefits, from blood pressure management to its impact on metabolic health, including diabetes and heart disease. But this isn't just a science textbook; it's a practical guide. We'll dive into the core components of the diet, discussing which foods to embrace, which to avoid, and how to ensure your meals are both nutritious and satisfying.

Phases are integral to the Rice Diet, providing a structured approach that eases you into this new way of eating. From detoxification and initial weight loss to transition and maintenance, each phase is designed to build upon the last, offering a clear path to long-term health. This phased approach ensures that the changes you make are sustainable, setting the foundation for a lifetime of wellness.

Implementing the Rice Diet is where theory meets practice. It's one thing to understand the principles; it's another to live them. This handbook offers practical tips for meal planning and preparation, managing hunger and cravings, and navigating the challenges of dining out and social events. It's about finding joy in the food you eat and peace in the choices you make.

Breakfast, lunch, dinner, snacks, sides, desserts, beverages—this book is packed with meal ideas that cater to every taste and need. Whether you're a fan of savory breakfasts or sweet treats, there's something here for everyone. These recipes are not just about adhering to dietary guidelines; they're about celebrating food and its ability to heal and delight.

And because we know that change can be daunting, we've included a 21-day meal plan to get you started. This plan is more than just a schedule of meals; it's a blueprint for success, offering a taste of the variety and satisfaction that the Rice Diet can bring to your life.

As you embark on this journey, remember: there will be challenges. There will be days when the old ways seem easier, more comforting. That's natural. Change is never easy, but it is possible. With this handbook as your guide, you have everything you need to make a lasting, positive change in your life.

So, let's begin this journey together. Here's to a healthier, happier you. Welcome to the Rice Diet.

Overview of the Rice Diet

The Rice Diet, in its essence, is simplicity married to nutrition, a dietary plan that champions the consumption of rice, fruits, vegetables, and legumes. It stands out in the vast sea of dietary regimens for its straightforward approach, focusing on whole, unprocessed foods that are low in sodium and rich in fiber. But to pigeonhole the Rice Diet as just another eating plan would be to overlook its transformative potential. This diet is more than a pathway to weight loss; it's a gateway to a healthier lifestyle, promising not just physical well-being but also a mental and emotional rejuvenation.

At its heart, the Rice Diet is built on the foundational belief that food can be medicine. By embracing a diet that is predominantly plant-based, participants can expect to see significant improvements in their overall health. The plan emphasizes the importance of simplicity, making it accessible to everyone, regardless of their culinary skills or knowledge about nutrition. Rice, the staple of the diet, is chosen for its versatility, digestibility, and the comforting satisfaction it provides. When combined with a colorful array of fruits and vegetables, as well as the protein and fiber from beans and legumes, the Rice Diet becomes a holistic nutritional powerhouse.

The structure of the Rice Diet is such that it encourages participants to eat in a mindful, deliberate manner. It promotes the idea of eating to fullness but not to excess, focusing on nutrient-dense foods that provide energy and promote satiety without the burden of excessive calories. This approach to eating can help address some of the root causes of overeating and weight gain, such as emotional eating and a reliance on processed foods.

One of the key features of the Rice Diet is its low sodium content. In a world where high-sodium diets are the norm, this diet offers a refreshing counterpoint that can have profound effects on health. By limiting sodium intake, participants can experience significant reductions in blood pressure, which in turn can decrease the risk of heart disease and stroke. This is particularly relevant in today's society, where such conditions are prevalent and often linked to dietary choices.

The Rice Diet also emphasizes the importance of hydration, encouraging the consumption of water and other non-caloric beverages to support kidney function and overall health. This focus on fluid intake is crucial, as hydration plays a key role in the body's ability to process nutrients and eliminate waste.

What sets the Rice Diet apart from other dietary plans is not just its components but its approach to health as a holistic concept. It's not merely about losing weight or lowering blood pressure; it's about creating a sustainable lifestyle that fosters well-being on every level. This diet encourages participants to look beyond the plate, considering how their food choices affect their health, their environment, and their world.

In embracing the Rice Diet, individuals are invited to embark on a journey of discovery, learning how simple, wholesome foods can transform their bodies and their lives. It's a diet that speaks to the power of simplicity, the value of mindfulness, and the profound impact that thoughtful food choices can have on our health.

As we delve deeper into the Rice Diet, it becomes clear that this is more than just a way of eating; it's a way of living. A life where food is both nourishment and pleasure, where eating is an act of self-care, and where each meal is a step towards a healthier, happier self.

Historical Background

The Rice Diet, with its roots firmly planted in the early 20th century, is more than just a dietary plan; it's a piece of medical history. Its origin story begins with Dr. Walter Kempner, a German physician and researcher, who joined Duke University in Durham, North Carolina, in 1939. Dr. Kempner's revolutionary approach to managing chronic illnesses through dietary intervention was, at the time, groundbreaking. His Rice Diet not only challenged prevailing medical norms but also laid the groundwork for understanding the profound connection between diet and health.

Dr. Kempner's primary objective was to address severe hypertension, kidney disease, and diabetes—conditions that were often considered irreversible and fatal in his time. The standard medical treatments available were largely ineffective and did not offer the promise of a long-term solution. It was within this context that Dr. Kempner began experimenting with a radical idea: Could a simple, controlled diet reverse these dire health conditions?

The Rice Diet was simple in its composition—white rice, fruit, juice, and sugar—yet revolutionary in its impact. This high-carbohydrate, low-fat, and low-sodium regimen was initially met with skepticism from the medical community. However, the results spoke for themselves. Patients not only lost weight but also showed remarkable improvements in blood pressure, kidney function, and blood sugar levels. The diet demonstrated an unprecedented ability to reverse the effects of chronic diseases, a feat that was nearly unheard of at the time.

What made the Rice Diet particularly innovative was Dr. Kempner's meticulous approach to patient care. Each participant in the program was closely monitored, with their dietary intake, physical activity, and health outcomes rigorously documented. This data-driven approach allowed Dr. Kempner to produce a wealth of evidence supporting the efficacy of the diet, contributing to its legitimacy and acceptance within the broader medical community.

The success of the Rice Diet at Duke University quickly garnered national attention, drawing patients from across the United States. Its popularity soared, and by the mid-20th century, the Rice Diet was not just a medical treatment but a cultural phenomenon. It represented a beacon of hope for those suffering from chronic illnesses, offering a non-invasive, diet-based path to recovery and health.

Over the decades, the Rice Diet evolved. While its core principles remained intact, modifications were made to incorporate a broader variety of foods and nutrients, reflecting advancements in nutritional science. The inclusion of vegetables, legumes, and eventually lean proteins and dairy, transformed the diet from a medical prescription into a lifestyle, one that could be adapted to meet the needs and preferences of a wider audience.

The legacy of Dr. Kempner and the Rice Diet is not merely in the diet itself but in the paradigm shift it prompted in the field of medicine. It underscored the power of dietary intervention in managing and reversing chronic diseases, paving the way for future research in nutritional science and holistic health. Today, the principles of the Rice Diet continue to influence dietary recommendations and health interventions, a testament to its enduring impact.

As we reflect on the historical background of the Rice Diet, it's important to recognize it as a pioneering effort that bridged the gap between nutrition and medicine. Its story is one of innovation, perseverance, and the relentless pursuit of health, offering valuable lessons for both healthcare professionals and individuals seeking a path to wellness.

Purpose and Goals

The Rice Diet, initially designed as a medical intervention for chronic diseases, has evolved into a comprehensive lifestyle choice with clear purposes and goals. At its inception, the primary aim was to combat hypertension, kidney disease, and diabetes, leveraging a diet-based approach to offer patients an alternative to the grim prognosis often associated with these conditions. However, as understanding and application of the diet expanded, so too did its objectives. Today, the Rice Diet serves multiple purposes, each centered on improving health and well-being.

Primary Objectives

1. **Health Restoration**: The foremost goal of the Rice Diet is health restoration. For individuals grappling with chronic conditions, the diet offers a pathway to not only manage but potentially reverse these ailments. By focusing on whole, nutrient-dense foods and limiting intake of sodium and unhealthy fats, the diet aims to recalibrate the body's natural mechanisms for maintaining health.

2. **Weight Management**: Weight loss is a natural byproduct of the Rice Diet, given its emphasis on low-calorie, high-fiber foods. For many, achieving and maintaining a healthy weight is a critical component of overall health, reducing the risk of diseases such as type 2 diabetes, heart disease, and certain cancers.

3. **Disease Prevention**: Beyond addressing existing health issues, the Rice Diet is geared towards disease prevention. The diet's nutrient profile—rich in vitamins, minerals, and antioxidants—supports the body's defense systems, helping to ward off illnesses before they start.

4. **Lifestyle Shift**: The diet encourages a holistic lifestyle shift, promoting not just changes in eating habits but also incorporating physical activity and mindfulness practices. This broader approach helps individuals achieve a balanced and healthy lifestyle that supports long-term well-being.

Secondary Objectives

- **Educational Aspect**: Part of the diet's goal is to educate individuals on the importance of nutrition and how dietary choices impact health. It aims to empower people with the knowledge and skills to make informed decisions about their diet and lifestyle.

- **Environmental Awareness**: By advocating for a plant-based diet, the Rice Diet also indirectly promotes environmental sustainability. It encourages a dietary pattern that is less resource-intensive, contributing to a lower environmental footprint.

- **Community and Support**: The Rice Diet fosters a sense of community among its followers, offering support and encouragement. This communal aspect is crucial, as it provides motivation and accountability, key factors in the success of any lifestyle change.

Long-Term Goals

The ultimate goal of the Rice Diet is not just temporary health improvements but the fostering of a sustainable, healthful lifestyle that can be maintained over the long term. It aims to instill habits that become second nature, ensuring that the benefits of the diet—improved health, weight management, disease prevention—are enduring.

Moreover, the Rice Diet seeks to influence the broader conversation around health and nutrition, advocating for a shift towards more mindful, health-conscious eating habits. It champions the idea that diet is not just about sustenance but about nourishment in the fullest sense—nourishing the body, mind, and spirit.

In conclusion, the Rice Diet is more than a set of dietary guidelines; it is a holistic approach to health and wellness. Its purpose and goals extend beyond the immediate benefits of weight loss and health improvement, aiming to transform lives through education, lifestyle changes, and community support. As we embark on this dietary journey, it's important to keep these objectives in mind, recognizing the profound impact that thoughtful, intentional eating can have on our overall quality of life.

THE SCIENCE BEHIND THE RICE DIET

Nutritional Foundations of the Rice Diet

The Rice Diet, renowned for its simplicity and effectiveness, is grounded in robust nutritional foundations that aim to promote optimal health, prevent and manage chronic diseases, and support sustainable weight management. This diet emphasizes the consumption of whole, unprocessed foods, primarily rice, fruits, vegetables, and legumes, forming a nutrient-dense foundation that supports the body's health and wellness needs. Here, we delve into the nutritional underpinnings of the Rice Diet, exploring its components, the rationale behind its food choices, and the scientific principles that underpin its health benefits.

Whole Grains: The Cornerstone

At the heart of the Rice Diet is rice, a staple grain consumed worldwide, revered for its versatility, digestibility, and nutritional profile. Whole grain rice, especially brown rice, is rich in complex carbohydrates, providing a steady source of energy, and is high in fiber, which aids in digestion and promotes satiety. Unlike refined grains, whole grains retain their bran and germ, ensuring a higher content of vitamins (such as B vitamins), minerals (including magnesium, selenium, and manganese), and phytochemicals, all of which play crucial roles in maintaining health.

Fruits and Vegetables: A Rainbow of Nutrients

Fruits and vegetables are pivotal in the Rice Diet, celebrated for their vast array of vitamins, minerals, antioxidants, and phytochemicals. These foods contribute not only to the diet's nutritional richness but also to its disease-fighting capabilities. The variety of colors in fruits and vegetables represents different nutrients and antioxidants, such as beta-carotene in orange produce, lycopene in red produce, and anthocyanins in blue and purple produce, each with unique health benefits. This diversity ensures comprehensive coverage of essential nutrients, supporting everything from immune function to heart health.

Legumes: Plant-Based Protein and Fiber

Legumes, including beans, lentils, and peas, are another cornerstone of the Rice Diet, providing high-quality plant-based protein, essential amino acids, and a wealth of fiber. This combination is crucial for maintaining muscle health, supporting digestive function, and regulating blood sugar levels. Legumes are also an excellent source of iron, potassium, and several B vitamins, contributing to a well-rounded, nutrient-dense dietary pattern.

Low Sodium: A Key to Cardiovascular Health

A hallmark of the Rice Diet is its low sodium content, a deliberate choice given the link between high sodium intake and hypertension, a major risk factor for cardiovascular disease. By limiting sodium, the diet promotes better blood pressure control and reduces strain on the cardiovascular system. The emphasis on whole foods naturally results in lower sodium intake, as processed and packaged foods are the primary sources of dietary sodium in many diets.

Limited Fats: Focusing on Quality over Quantity

While the Rice Diet is not strictly low-fat, it advocates for the consumption of healthy fats and limits saturated and trans fats. The inclusion of small amounts of nuts, seeds, and possibly fatty fish (for those who choose to include animal products) ensures the intake of essential fatty acids, including omega-3s, which are known for their anti-inflammatory properties and role in heart health.

Hydration and Fluid Intake

Hydration is another key aspect of the Rice Diet's nutritional foundation. Adequate fluid intake is essential for kidney function, digestion, and overall cellular health. The diet encourages drinking water and other low-calorie beverages to support the body's hydration needs, complementing the diet's solid food components.

Scientific Principles Supporting the Diet

The nutritional principles of the Rice Diet are supported by a wealth of scientific evidence highlighting the benefits of whole grains, a plant-based diet, reduced sodium intake, and adequate hydration. Studies have consistently shown that diets rich in fruits, vegetables, and whole grains, and low in processed foods and sodium, can lead to improvements in cardiovascular health, weight management, and metabolic function. The Rice Diet's focus on these principles makes it effective not only for disease management but also for promoting long-term health and well-being.

Health Benefits

The Rice Diet, with its emphasis on whole, plant-based foods, offers a multitude of health benefits that extend far beyond weight loss. This nutritionally rich diet impacts various aspects of health, contributing to cardiovascular health, improved metabolic function, and enhanced overall well-being. Here, we explore the myriad health benefits associated with the Rice Diet, underpinned by nutritional science and clinical research.

Cardiovascular Health

One of the most significant benefits of the Rice Diet is its positive impact on cardiovascular health. The diet's low sodium and low saturated fat content, coupled with its high fiber intake from whole grains, fruits, and vegetables, contribute to lower blood pressure and improved lipid profiles. These changes are instrumental in reducing the risk of heart disease, stroke, and other cardiovascular conditions. Research has consistently shown that diets rich in fiber and low in unhealthy fats can lead to reductions in LDL (bad) cholesterol and improvements in arterial function, highlighting the cardiovascular benefits of the Rice Diet.

Metabolic Health

The Rice Diet also offers considerable advantages for metabolic health, including blood sugar control and insulin sensitivity. The high fiber content of the diet slows the absorption of sugar into the bloodstream, preventing spikes in blood glucose levels and supporting overall glycemic control. This is particularly beneficial for individuals with diabetes or those at risk of developing the condition. Furthermore, the diet's plant-based nature and low glycemic index foods can enhance insulin sensitivity, making it easier for the body to manage blood sugar levels efficiently.

Weight Management

Weight loss and management are key outcomes for many adherents of the Rice Diet. By emphasizing low-calorie, nutrient-dense foods, the diet naturally leads to a reduction in calorie intake without sacrificing satiety or nutritional adequacy. This can result in a steady, sustainable weight loss, which is crucial for the prevention and management of obesity-related conditions, including type 2 diabetes, hypertension, and certain forms of cancer. The inclusion of a variety of whole foods also ensures that the body receives a balanced array of nutrients, supporting overall health during weight loss efforts.

The low sodium content of the Rice Diet is particularly beneficial for kidney health. High sodium intake is associated with increased blood pressure, which can strain the kidneys and exacerbate conditions such as chronic kidney disease (CKD). By reducing sodium intake, the Rice Diet can help lower blood pressure and alleviate the burden on the kidneys, potentially slowing the progression of CKD and supporting overall kidney function.

Digestive Health

The high fiber content of the Rice Diet also supports digestive health. Fiber aids in maintaining regular bowel movements and can help prevent constipation, diverticulosis, and other gastrointestinal disorders. Additionally, a diet rich in fruits and vegetables provides prebiotics, which feed beneficial gut bacteria and contribute to a healthy microbiome, further enhancing digestive wellness.

Reduction in Inflammation

The anti-inflammatory properties of many foods included in the Rice Diet, such as fruits, vegetables, whole grains, and legumes, contribute to a reduction in systemic inflammation. Chronic inflammation is a key factor in the development of many diseases, including heart disease, diabetes, and cancer. By adopting a diet that is rich in anti-inflammatory foods, individuals can potentially lower their risk of these conditions.

Overall Well-Being

Beyond specific physical health benefits, the Rice Diet can also contribute to improved mental health and well-being. Nutrient-dense diets have been linked to better mood, increased energy levels, and improved sleep quality, all of which are essential for overall quality of life.

Blood Pressure Management

Hypertension, or high blood pressure, is a prevalent condition that significantly increases the risk of heart disease, stroke, and kidney problems. The Rice Diet's efficacy in managing blood pressure lies in its fundamental principles: a low sodium intake, a high intake of fruits and vegetables, and a focus on whole grains and legumes. Each of these components plays a vital role in regulating blood pressure levels, offering a natural, diet-based solution to a condition often managed with medication.

Low Sodium Intake

A cornerstone of the Rice Diet is its low sodium content. Excessive sodium consumption is a well-known risk factor for hypertension. The Rice Diet addresses this directly by significantly reducing the intake of salt and processed foods, which are primary sources of dietary sodium. By emphasizing whole, natural foods, the diet naturally limits sodium intake, helping to lower blood pressure. Scientific research supports the link between reduced sodium intake and decreased blood pressure, making this aspect of the Rice Diet particularly effective for hypertension management.

Potassium-Rich Foods

The diet also focuses on the consumption of potassium-rich foods, such as fruits and vegetables. Potassium helps balance the effects of sodium in the body and eases tension in the blood vessel walls, both of which are beneficial for lowering blood pressure. Foods like bananas, spinach, sweet potatoes, and tomatoes are staples in the Rice Diet, providing ample potassium to support blood pressure management. The inclusion of these foods aligns with the Dietary

Approaches to Stop Hypertension (DASH) diet principles, which are also known for their blood pressure-lowering effects.

Plant-Based Diet and Blood Pressure

Adopting a plant-based diet, as the Rice Diet suggests, has been associated with lower blood pressure. Plant-based diets are typically lower in fat and calories and higher in fiber, which can positively affect body weight, another important factor in blood pressure control. Moreover, the antioxidants and phytochemicals found in fruits, vegetables, and whole grains can improve vascular health, further contributing to blood pressure reduction.

Weight Loss and Blood Pressure

Weight loss is a direct benefit of the Rice Diet, given its low-calorie yet nutrient-dense food choices. Excess body weight is a significant risk factor for hypertension, and even modest weight loss can have a meaningful impact on reducing blood pressure levels. The Rice Diet facilitates weight loss through its emphasis on satiety and nutrition, helping individuals achieve and maintain a healthy weight, which in turn supports healthy blood pressure levels.

Scientific Evidence and Clinical Studies

Clinical studies and research have consistently shown the benefits of dietary changes on blood pressure control. The Rice Diet's approach mirrors the findings of these studies, offering a practical and effective way to manage hypertension through food. By adhering to the diet's guidelines, individuals can experience significant improvements in blood pressure, often within just a few weeks.

Integrating the Rice Diet into Hypertension Management

For those with hypertension, integrating the Rice Diet into their lifestyle can be a powerful tool in managing their condition. It's important, however, to approach this dietary change under the guidance of a healthcare professional, especially for individuals already on blood pressure medication, as adjustments may be necessary.

Kidney Health

The Rice Diet's positive effects on kidney health are rooted in its foundational principles, particularly its low sodium content, emphasis on whole foods, and avoidance of processed and fatty foods. Kidneys play a crucial role in filtering waste products, balancing bodily fluids, and regulating blood pressure. A diet that supports kidney function can significantly impact the prevention and management of kidney-related issues.

Low Sodium Intake and Kidney Function

High sodium intake is a well-known risk factor for hypertension, which in turn can put additional strain on the kidneys, exacerbating conditions such as chronic kidney disease (CKD). The Rice Diet's low sodium approach helps mitigate this risk, reducing the burden on kidneys by maintaining healthier blood pressure levels. This aspect of the diet not only aids in blood pressure management but also directly benefits kidney health by minimizing the kidneys' workload in filtering and excreting sodium.

Protein Moderation

The traditional Rice Diet also focuses on moderate protein intake, primarily from plant sources. High protein diets, especially those rich in animal protein, can increase the kidneys' workload, potentially harming individuals with compromised kidney function. By emphasizing plant-based protein sources, the Rice Diet ensures adequate protein intake without overburdening the kidneys, making it a viable option for individuals seeking to maintain or improve kidney health.

Antioxidant-Rich Foods

Fruits, vegetables, and whole grains, staples of the Rice Diet, are rich in antioxidants and anti-inflammatory compounds. These nutrients play a vital role in protecting the kidneys from damage by neutralizing harmful free radicals and reducing inflammation. Chronic inflammation can contribute to the progression of kidney disease, and a diet high in antioxidants can help counteract these effects, supporting renal health.

Hydration and Kidney Health

Adequate hydration is essential for kidney function, as it helps the kidneys filter waste from the blood and excrete it in the urine. The Rice Diet encourages a high intake of water and other hydrating fluids, complementing its solid food components and supporting the body's natural detoxification processes through the kidneys. Proper hydration is crucial for preventing kidney stones and other renal complications.

Impact on Kidney Disease

For individuals with CKD or at risk of developing kidney disease, dietary modifications like those proposed by the Rice Diet can be particularly beneficial. By reducing sodium intake, moderating protein consumption, and increasing the intake of fruits and vegetables, the diet can help manage CKD's progression and alleviate symptoms.

Weight Loss and Metabolic Improvements

Caloric Density and Nutrient Richness

The Rice Diet is characterized by foods with low caloric density but high nutrient content. Whole grains like brown rice, fruits, vegetables, and legumes fill you up without contributing excessive calories. This approach encourages eating larger volumes of food that satisfy hunger, making it easier to maintain a calorie deficit without feeling deprived. The fiber in these foods adds to the feeling of fullness and slows digestion, which helps control appetite and prevent overeating.

Natural Reduction in Calorie Intake

By focusing on whole, plant-based foods and limiting processed foods, fats, and sweets, the Rice Diet naturally reduces overall calorie intake. Without the need to meticulously count calories, individuals can lose weight through simple dietary adjustments. This ease of adherence is a key factor in the diet's effectiveness for long-term weight management.

Impact on Metabolic Health

The Rice Diet not only aids in weight loss but also significantly improves metabolic markers, including blood sugar levels, lipid profiles, and insulin sensitivity. The diet's high fiber content and low glycemic index foods contribute to more stable blood sugar levels, reducing the risk of insulin resistance—a precursor to type 2 diabetes.

Metabolic Improvements

Enhanced Insulin Sensitivity

A diet rich in whole grains, legumes, and vegetables, as advocated by the Rice Diet, has been associated with improvements in insulin sensitivity. This is crucial for metabolic health, as improved insulin sensitivity helps the body use glucose more effectively, lowering blood sugar levels and reducing the risk of diabetes.

Lowering of Blood Lipids

The Rice Diet can lead to significant reductions in cholesterol and triglyceride levels, thanks to its low intake of saturated fats and high intake of fiber. Soluble fiber, found in fruits, vegetables, and legumes, binds cholesterol in the digestive system, facilitating its excretion and thus lowering blood cholesterol levels. These changes can reduce the risk of heart disease and stroke, contributing to overall cardiovascular health.

Prevention and Management of Type 2 Diabetes

By promoting a stable, slow release of glucose into the bloodstream, the Rice Diet can prevent the typical blood sugar spikes and crashes associated with refined carbohydrate consumption. This steady glycemic control is beneficial for preventing type 2 diabetes in at-risk individuals and managing the condition in those already diagnosed.

Practical Tips for Maximizing Weight Loss and Metabolic Benefits

Portion Control and Mindful Eating

While the Rice Diet promotes eating healthily, attention to portion sizes and practicing mindful eating can enhance weight loss efforts. Listening to hunger cues, eating slowly, and enjoying meals without distractions can prevent overeating and contribute to a healthier relationship with food.

Regular Physical Activity

Incorporating regular physical activity into the lifestyle changes recommended by the Rice Diet can accelerate weight loss and further improve metabolic health. Exercise boosts metabolism, increases muscle mass, and helps burn calories, complementing the diet's effects.

Consistency and Patience

Sustainable weight loss and metabolic improvements require time and consistency. The Rice Diet emphasizes long-term lifestyle changes over quick fixes. Patience and persistence are key to realizing the full benefits of the diet.

Monitoring Progress

Keeping track of progress, whether through regular weigh-ins, body measurements, or monitoring blood glucose and lipid levels, can provide motivation and insight into how well the diet is working for an individual's specific health goals.

Impact on Diabetes and Heart Disease

Impact on Diabetes

Diabetes, particularly type 2 diabetes, is closely linked to dietary habits, body weight, and metabolic health. The Rice Diet's low-fat, high-fiber content, and focus on whole, unprocessed foods make it an effective tool for managing and preventing diabetes.

Improved Glycemic Control

The high fiber content of the Rice Diet plays a crucial role in blood sugar regulation. Dietary fiber slows the absorption of sugar into the bloodstream, preventing spikes in blood glucose levels after meals. This steady glycemic control is crucial for managing diabetes and reducing the risk of developing the disease.

Weight Management

Obesity is a significant risk factor for type 2 diabetes. The Rice Diet, through its emphasis on nutrient-dense, low-calorie foods, facilitates weight loss and helps maintain a healthy body weight. This weight management is key to preventing insulin resistance, a precursor to diabetes.

Enhanced Insulin Sensitivity

The diet's plant-based nature and low intake of saturated fats improve insulin sensitivity. Improved insulin sensitivity allows the body to use glucose more efficiently, reducing the burden on the pancreas to produce insulin and lowering blood sugar levels.

Impact on Heart Disease

Heart disease remains a leading cause of morbidity and mortality worldwide. The Rice Diet combats several risk factors associated with heart disease, including hypertension, high cholesterol, and obesity.

Blood Pressure Reduction

As previously discussed, the low sodium content of the Rice Diet, coupled with its emphasis on fruits and vegetables rich in potassium, helps lower blood pressure. Hypertension is a major risk factor for heart disease, and its management is vital for cardiovascular health.

Cholesterol and Lipid Levels

The Rice Diet's low intake of saturated fats and cholesterol, and its high fiber content, contribute to lower blood cholesterol levels. Specifically, it reduces LDL (bad) cholesterol, which is implicated in plaque formation within the arteries, leading to atherosclerosis and heart disease.

Weight Loss and Cardiovascular Health

Excess weight, particularly around the abdomen, increases the risk of heart disease. The Rice Diet's effectiveness in promoting weight loss and reducing body fat contributes to a lower risk of cardiovascular conditions, including heart failure and stroke.

Implementing the Rice Diet for Diabetes and Heart Disease Managements

Personalization

While the Rice Diet provides a foundation, personalization based on individual health status, preferences, and goals is crucial. Consulting with healthcare professionals can ensure the diet meets nutritional needs and effectively addresses specific health concerns.

Monitoring and Adjustment

Regular monitoring of blood sugar levels, blood pressure, and lipid profiles can help gauge the diet's effectiveness and guide adjustments. This ongoing assessment ensures the dietary approach remains aligned with health objectives.

Holistic Approach

Combining the Rice Diet with other lifestyle modifications, such as regular physical activity, stress management, and smoking cessation, maximizes the benefits for diabetes and heart disease prevention and management.

Comparative Analysis with Other Diets

Comparison with the Mediterranean Diet

The Mediterranean Diet is renowned for its heart-healthy benefits, emphasizing fruits, vegetables, whole grains, olive oil, fish, and moderate wine consumption. Both the Mediterranean and Rice Diets prioritize plant-based foods and limit red meat, reflecting a shared focus on reducing heart disease risk and promoting overall health. However, the Rice Diet is more restrictive in sodium intake and emphasizes rice as a staple, distinguishing it from the Mediterranean Diet's broader inclusion of whole grains and more significant emphasis on healthy fats from olive oil and nuts.

Comparison with the DASH Diet

The Dietary Approaches to Stop Hypertension (DASH) Diet is specifically designed to combat high blood pressure, featuring a balanced intake of fruits, vegetables, whole grains, lean protein, and low-fat dairy, while limiting sodium, red meat, and added sugars. The Rice Diet and DASH Diet share similar objectives, especially regarding sodium reduction and the promotion of fruits and vegetables. However, the Rice Diet places a stronger emphasis on rice and is generally lower in protein, particularly animal protein, than the DASH Diet.

Comparison with Low-Carb and Keto Diets

Low-carb and ketogenic diets reduce carbohydrate intake to varying degrees to promote weight loss and improve metabolic health. These diets contrast sharply with the Rice Diet, which is based on high-carbohydrate, low-fat principles. While low-carb and keto diets focus on high fat and protein intake, the Rice Diet emphasizes complex carbohydrates from whole grains, fruits, and vegetables. The Rice Diet's approach is less about inducing ketosis and more about providing a balanced, nutrient-dense eating pattern that supports long-term health and weight management.

Comparison with Plant-Based Diets

Plant-based diets, including vegan and vegetarian diets, eliminate or significantly reduce animal products, focusing instead on fruits, vegetables, grains, nuts, and seeds. The Rice Diet shares similarities with plant-based diets in its emphasis on vegetables, grains, and legumes. However, the Rice Diet is not inherently vegetarian or vegan, as it allows for the inclusion of small amounts of animal protein. The primary focus on rice as a staple also sets it apart from other plant-based diets, which may include a wider variety of grains.

Nutritional Balance and Flexibility

One of the Rice Diet's strengths is its simplicity and the emphasis on unprocessed foods, which can contribute to improved health outcomes. However, its restrictive nature and heavy emphasis on rice may not provide the dietary variety needed for optimal nutritional balance compared to diets like the Mediterranean or DASH diets, which offer a broader range of food choices and nutrients.

Sustainability and Long-Term Adherence

Sustainability is a crucial factor in the effectiveness of any diet. The Rice Diet's restrictive nature may pose challenges for long-term adherence for some individuals, compared to more flexible approaches like the Mediterranean Diet, which is often celebrated for its palatability and ease of integration into various lifestyles.

FOODS TO INCLUDE CHARTS IN THE RICE DIET

Rice Varieties

Food (Rice Variety)	Portion Size	Calories	Carbohydrates (g)	Protein (g)
Arborio Rice, Cooked	1 cup (157g)	194	42	4
Bamboo Rice, Cooked	1 cup (150g)	160	34	3.5
Basmati Rice, Cooked	1 cup (163g)	210	45.6	4.4
Bhutanese Red Rice, Cooked	1 cup (158g)	210	45	4
Black Japonica Rice, Cooked	1 cup (180g)	200	43	6
Black Rice, Cooked	1 cup (180g)	160	34	5
Blue Rice, Cooked	1 cup (150g)	210	45	4
Brown Rice, Long Grain, Cooked	1 cup (195g)	248	51.7	5.5
Calrose Rice, Cooked	1 cup (158g)	200	44	4

Camargue Red Rice, Cooked	1 cup (158g)	215	45	4
Carnaroli Rice, Cooked	1 cup (160g)	200	44	4
Chak Hao Rice, Cooked	1 cup (158g)	200	45	4
Colusari Red Rice, Cooked	1 cup (160g)	200	45	4
Egyptian Rice, Cooked	1 cup (150g)	210	45	4.5
Forbidden Rice, Cooked	1 cup (150g)	200	44	6
Glutinous Black Rice, Cooked	1 cup (180g)	180	40	4
Gobindobhog Rice, Cooked	1 cup (158g)	210	44	4
Italian Red Rice, Cooked	1 cup (180g)	200	45	4
Japonica Rice, Cooked	1 cup (150g)	210	46	4.5
Jasmine Rice, Cooked	1 cup (158g)	238	52	4.2
Kalijira Rice, Cooked	1 cup (150g)	200	44	4
Long Grain Brown Rice, Cooked	1 cup (195g)	216	45	5

Madagascar Pink Rice, Cooked	1 cup (160g)	200	45	4
Matta Rice, Cooked	1 cup (160g)	220	45	5
Medium Grain Brown Rice, Cooked	1 cup (195g)	218	46	4.5
Mochi Rice, Cooked	1 cup (180g)	220	49	4.5
Parboiled Rice, Cooked	1 cup (175g)	194	41	5
Patna Rice, Cooked	1 cup (158g)	200	44	4
Pink Rice, Cooked	1 cup (150g)	200	45	5
Ponni Rice, Cooked	1 cup (160g)	206	45	4
Puffed Rice	1 cup (14g)	56	12.5	1
Purple Thai Rice, Cooked	1 cup (180g)	240	50	5
Red Cargo Rice, Cooked	1 cup (180g)	210	45	5
Red Rice, Cooked	1 cup (202g)	216	45	5
Rice Flakes, Cooked	1 cup (145g)	130	28	2.5

Rosematta Rice, Cooked	1 cup (160g)	194	42	4
Short Grain Brown Rice, Cooked	1 cup (195g)	215	44	5
Sona Masoori Rice, Cooked	1 cup (160g)	200	44	4
Sprouted Brown Rice, Cooked	1 cup (160g)	212	46	5
Sticky Rice, Cooked	1 cup (200g)	169	37	3.5
Sushi Rice, Cooked	1 cup (158g)	210	46	4
Sweet Brown Rice, Cooked	1 cup (190g)	230	49	5
Texmati Rice, Cooked	1 cup (150g)	190	40	4
Thai Black Sticky Rice, Cooked	1 cup (180g)	160	34	3.5
Valencia Rice, Cooked	1 cup (160g)	190	42	4
Vialone Nano Rice, Cooked	1 cup (160g)	210	46	4
Wehani Rice, Cooked	1 cup (160g)	170	36	4
Wehani Rice, Cooked	1 cup (160g)	170	35	4

White Rice, Long Grain, Cooked	1 cup (158g)	205	44.5	4.3
Wild Rice, Cooked	1 cup (164g)	166	35	6.5

Fruits and Vegetables

Food (Fruit/Vegetable)	Portion Size	Calories	Key Vitamin	Fiber (g)
Apple	1 medium (182g)	95	Vitamin C	4.4
Asparagus	1 cup (134g)	27	Vitamin K	2.8
Avocado	1/2 fruit (100g)	160	Vitamin E	6.7
Avocado	1/2 fruit (100g)	160	Vitamin E	6.7
Banana	1 medium (118g)	105	Vitamin B6	3.1
Banana	1 medium (118g)	105	Vitamin B6	3.1
Beetroot	1 cup (136g)	58	Fiber	3.8
Bell Pepper	1 cup (149g)	25	Vitamin C	1.7
Blackberries	1 cup (144g)	62	Vitamin C	7.6
Blueberries	1 cup (148g)	84	Vitamin C	3.6

Blueberries	1 cup (148g)	84	Vitamin C	3.6
Broccoli	1 cup (91g)	31	Vitamin C	2.4
Broccoli	1 cup (91g)	31	Vitamin C	2.4
Brussels Sprouts	1 cup (88g)	38	Vitamin K	3.3
Cantaloupe	1 cup (160g)	53	Vitamin A	1.4
Carrot	1 medium (61g)	25	Vitamin A	1.7
Carrot	1 medium (61g)	25	Vitamin A	1.7
Cauliflower	1 cup (100g)	25	Vitamin C	2
Cherries	1 cup (138g)	87	Vitamin C	2.5
Cucumber	1 cup (104g)	16	Vitamin K	0.5
Eggplant	1 cup (99g)	20	Fiber	2.8
Grapes	1 cup (151g)	104	Vitamin K	1.4
Kale	1 cup (67g)	33	Vitamin K	2.5
Kale	1 cup (67g)	33	Vitamin K	2.5
Kiwi	1 medium (69g)	42	Vitamin C	2.1

Leek	1 cup (89g)	54	Vitamin K	1.6
Mango	1 cup (165g)	99	Vitamin C	2.6
Nectarines	1 medium (142g)	63	Vitamin C	2.4
Okra	1 cup (100g)	33	Vitamin K	3.2
Orange	1 medium (131g)	62	Vitamin C	3.1
Papaya	1 cup (145g)	62	Vitamin C	2.5
Peaches	1 medium (150g)	59	Vitamin C	2
Pear	1 medium (178g)	101	Fiber	5.5
Peas	1 cup (160g)	117	Vitamin K	7.4
Pineapple	1 cup (165g)	82	Vitamin C	2.3
Pomegranate	1 cup (174g)	144	Vitamin C	7
Pumpkin	1 cup (116g)	30	Vitamin A	0.6
Radish	1 cup (116g)	19	Vitamin C	1.9
Raspberries	1 cup (123g)	64	Vitamin C	8
Spinach	1 cup (30g)	7	Vitamin K	0.7

Spinach	1 cup (30g)	7	Vitamin K	0.7
Strawberries	1 cup (152g)	49	Vitamin C	3
Sweet Potato	1 medium (114g)	103	Vitamin A	4
Sweet Potato	1 medium (114g)	103	Vitamin A	4
Tomato	1 medium (123g)	22	Vitamin C	1.5
Tomato	1 medium (123g)	22	Vitamin C	1.5
Turnip	1 cup (130g)	36	Vitamin C	3.1
Watermelon	1 cup (154g)	46	Vitamin C	0.6
Zucchini	1 cup (124g)	20	Vitamin C	1.4

Additional Plant-Based Foods

Food	Portion Size	Calories	Protein (g)	Fiber (g)
Almonds, raw	1 oz (28g)	161	6	3.5
Amaranth, cooked	1 cup (246g)	251	9.3	5.2
Artichoke, cooked	1 medium (120g)	64	3.5	7
Barley, cooked	1 cup (157g)	193	3.5	6
Beet Greens, cooked	1 cup (144g)	39	3.7	4.2
Black Beans, cooked	1 cup (172g)	227	15.2	15
Brown Rice, cooked	1 cup (195g)	216	5	3.5
Brussels Sprouts, cooked	1 cup (156g)	56	4	4.1
Buckwheat, cooked	1 cup (168g)	155	5.7	4.5
Bulgur, cooked	1 cup (182g)	151	5.6	8.2
Cashews, raw	1 oz (28g)	157	5	0.9
Chia Seeds	1 oz (28g)	138	4.7	9.8
Chia Seeds	1 oz (28g)	138	4.7	9.8
Chickpeas, cooked	1 cup (164g)	269	14.5	12.5
Edamame, cooked	1 cup (155g)	188	18.5	8.1

Farro, cooked	1 cup (174g)	200	8	7.5
Flaxseeds	1 oz (28g)	150	5.1	7.6
Freekeh, cooked	1 cup (140g)	132	4.3	4.5
Green Peas, cooked	1 cup (160g)	125	8.2	8.8
Hemp Seeds	1 oz (28g)	155	9	1
Kale, raw	1 cup (67g)	33	2.9	1.3
Kidney Beans, cooked	1 cup (177g)	225	15.3	11
Lentils, cooked	1 cup (198g)	230	18	15.6
Mung Beans, cooked	1 cup (202g)	212	14.2	15.4
Navy Beans, cooked	1 cup (182g)	255	15	11.6
Oatmeal, cooked	1 cup (234g)	158	6	4
Peanut Butter	2 tbsp (32g)	188	8	2.6
Peanuts, roasted	1 oz (28g)	166	7	2.3
Pinto Beans, cooked	1 cup (171g)	245	15.4	15.4
Pistachios, raw	1 oz (28g)	159	5.7	3
Pumpkin Seeds, roasted	1 oz (28.35g)	126	5.3	5.2
Quinoa, cooked	1 cup (185g)	222	8	5.2

Seitan	3 oz (85g)	104	21	0.5
Sorghum, cooked	1 cup (192g)	214	5.4	6.3
Spirulina, dried	1 tbsp (7g)	20	4	0.1
Sunflower Seeds, roasted	1 oz (28g)	164	5.5	2.4
Sweet Corn, cooked	1 cup (164g)	177	5.4	4.6
Swiss Chard, cooked	1 cup (175g)	35	3.3	3.7
Tempeh	1 cup (166g)	320	31	6
Tofu, firm	100g	144	16.7	2
Walnuts, raw	1 oz (28g)	185	4.3	1.9

FOODS TO AVOID CHARTS IN THE RICE DIET

High-Sodium Foods

Food Item	Portion Size	Sodium (mg)	Calories	Total Fat (g)
Anchovies	1 oz	1100-1500	40-60	2-3
Bacon	2 slices	300-400	80-100	7-10
Bagels with Cream Cheese	1 item	500-700	250-350	6-9
Beef Jerky	1 oz	600-1000	70-120	1-5
Biscuits	1 biscuit	400-500	150-250	6-10
Blue Cheese	1 oz	325-500	100-110	8-10
Bottled Tomato Sauce	1/2 cup	400-600	70-90	1-3
Caesar Salad Dressing	2 tbsp	300-500	150-200	15-18
Canned Baked Beans	1/2 cup	550-750	120-180	0.5-2
Canned Chili	1 cup	800-1200	200-300	10-15
Canned Soup	1 cup	800-1300	100-200	3-9
Canned Tuna in Brine	2 oz	250-350	50-70	0.5-1
Canned Vegetables	1/2 cup	200-500	20-60	0-1
Cheese	1 oz	200-500	100-120	9-11
Chicken Nuggets	6 nuggets	600-900	270-330	17-20

Clam Chowder	1 cup	800-1000	200-300	10-15
Corned Beef	3 oz	900-1100	210-250	16-18
Cottage Cheese	1/2 cup	350-450	90-110	2-5
Fast Food Burgers	1 burger	600-1300	250-600	10-40
Flavored Rice Mixes	1 cup cooked	750-1250	210-310	0.5-4
French Fries	3 oz	250-450	220-300	10-15
Frozen Pizza	1 slice	500-800	250-450	10-20
Gravy	1/4 cup	300-500	30-70	2-5
Hot Dogs	1 hot dog	500-700	150-250	14-16
Instant Mashed Potatoes	1 cup	500-750	200-250	1-5
Instant Noodles	1 package	800-1500	180-380	7-14
Ketchup	1 tbsp	150-200	15-20	0
Mustard	1 tsp	55-120	55-120	0.2-0.5
Olives	1 oz	300-400	40-50	4-5
Pickles	1 medium	800-1100	15-30	0-0.5
Pretzels	1 oz	300-500	100-150	1-2
Processed Deli Meats	2 slices	600-1200	70-120	2-9
Ramen	1 package	1500-2000	380-500	14-18
Salad Dressings	2 tbsp	200-500	100-200	10-20
Salted Butter	1 tbsp	90-150	100-110	11-12
Salted Caramel Desserts	1 piece	200-400	250-350	15-Oct
Salted Caramel Ice Cream	1/2 cup	100-200	180-250	10-15
Salted Nuts	1 oz	100-300	160-200	14-18
Salted Popcorn	1 oz	100-300	110-130	6-8

Salted Pretzel Chocolate Bars	1 bar	200-400	200-300	10-15
Sardines in Canned Saltwater	2 oz	300-500	100-200	5-10
Sauerkraut	1/2 cup	460-750	20-40	0-1
Smoked Salmon	2 oz	600-1200	70-100	2-5
Snack Crackers	1 oz	200-300	120-150	5-7
Soy Sauce	1 tbsp	900-1100	010-015	0
Spaghetti with Meat Sauce	1 cup	400-800	200-300	5-10
Table Salt	1 tsp	2300	0	0
Teriyaki Sauce	1 tbsp	690-900	15-25	0
Tortilla Chips	1 oz	120-180	140-160	7-9
Tuna Salad	1/2 cup	300-600	200-300	10-20

Fatty Foods

Food Item	Portion Size	Calories (approx.)	Total Fat (g)	Saturated Fat (g)
Bagels	1 large	310	1.5	0.3
Beef Jerky	1 oz	116	7	3
Biscuits	1 medium	212	11	6
Buffalo Wings	3 wings	216	15	4.5
Canned Coconut Milk	1 cup	445	48	43
Canned Soup (Creamy)	1 cup	180	9	6
Caramel Latte	16 oz	250	7	4.5
Cheddar Cheese	1 oz	113	9	6
Cheesecake	1 slice	401	28	18
Chocolate Bar	1.55 oz	220	13	8
Chocolate Chip Cookies	4 cookies	260	14	6
Coconut Oil	1 tablespoon	121	14	12
Creamy Salad Dressing	2 tablespoons	140	15	2.5
Croissants	1 medium	235	12	7
Deep-Fried Foods	1 serving	340-500	22-30	5-10
Fettuccine Alfredo	1 cup	660	47	28
Fried Fish	1 fillet	205	11	2.3
Full-Fat Cheese	1 oz	110	9	6
Granola Bars	1 bar	118	6	2.5

Heavy Cream	1 cup	821	88	2-24
Hot Dogs	1 hot dog	150	13	4.5
Lard	1 tablespoon	115	13	5
Lasagna	1 slice	350	17	7
Macaroni and Cheese	1 cup	310	12	7
Mayonnaise	1 tablespoon	94	10	1.6
Milk Chocolate	1 oz	150	8.5	5
Muffins	1 medium	410	19	3.5
Nachos with Cheese	1 serving	346	18	6
Olive Oil	1 tablespoon	119	14	2
Pancakes with Syrup	2 pancakes	520	12	1-2
Peanut Butter (Creamy)	2 tablespoons	188	16	3.4
Pecan Pie	1 slice	503	27	14
Pork Rinds	1 oz	154	9	3.2
Quiche	1 slice	640	45	18
Ribs (Pork)	3 oz	232	18	6.5
Salami	1 oz	110	9	3.5
Sausage	2 links	140	12	4.2
Sour Cream	2 tablespoons	60	5	3.5
Steak (Ribeye)	3 oz	207	13	5
Sugar-Sweetened Beverages	12 oz	150-200	0	0
Sweetened Yogurt	1 cup	200	3.5	2.2

Tacos (Beef)	2 tacos	290	17	6
Tiramisu	1 slice	240	11	6.5
Tortilla Chips	1 oz	138	7	1.2
Whipped Cream	1 cup	154	13	8.4
White Bread	1 slice	66	0.8	0.2

Processed and Refined Foods

Food	Portion Size	Sodium (mg)	Fats (g)	Sugars (g)
Artificially Sweetened Beverages	1 can (355ml)	40	0	0 (artificial)
BBQ Sauce	2 tbsp (28g)	280	0	11
Biscuits	1 biscuit (60g)	490	22	3
Bottled Salad Dressings	2 tbsp (30ml)	280	15	2
Boxed Macaroni and Cheese	1 cup (70g)	570	3.5	6
Breakfast Cereals (High Sugar)	1 cup (30-60g)	200	1	12
Candy Bars	1 bar (50g)	75	9	24
Canned Baked Beans in Sauce	1/2 cup (130g)	550	0.5	12
Canned Chili	1 cup (247g)	1300	7	6
Canned Fruit in Heavy Syrup	1/2 cup (122g)	10	0	23
Canned Pasta Sauce	1/2 cup (128g)	480	3.5	12
Canned Soups	1 cup (240ml)	940	5	6

Cereal Bars	1 bar (40g)	120	4	24
Cream-filled Pastries	1 pastry (60g)	170	10	16
Deli Meats	2 oz (56g)	600	5	2
Doughnuts	1 medium (85g)	200	15	23
Energy Drinks	1 can (250ml)	200	0	27
Fast Food Burgers	1 burger (200g)	490	24	9
Flavored Coffee Creamers	1 tbsp (15ml)	25	1.5	5
Flavored Gelatin	1/2 cup (120g)	85	0	18
Flavored Popcorn	1 oz (28g)	150	9	0
Flavored Potato Chips	1 oz (28g)	150	10	1
Flavored Water	1 bottle (500ml)	0	0	15
Flavored Yogurts	1 cup (245g)	100	3.5	47
French Fries	1 medium (117g)	246	13	0.3
Fried Chicken	1 piece (150g)	1200	15	0
Frozen Dinners	1 package (255g)	800	12	5
Frozen Pizza	1 slice (107g)	700	12	4
Fruit Snacks	1 package (23g)	10	0	11
Ice Cream	1/2 cup (68g)	45	7	14
Instant Noodles	1 package (85g)	830	14	2
Instant Oatmeal Packets	1 packet (45g)	260	2	12
Instant Pudding Mix	1/2 cup (prepared) (120g)	350	2.5	20
Ketchup	1 tbsp (17g)	160	0	4
Margarine	1 tbsp (14g)	160	11	0
Milk Chocolate	1 oz (28g)	20	9	15
Packaged Cupcakes	1 cupcake (53g)	150	5	35
Packaged Muffins	1 muffin (113g)	400	17	24
Packaged Snack Cakes	1 cake (42g)	180	9	20

Potato Chips	1 oz (28g)	170	10	0.5
Pre-packaged Sandwiches	1 sandwich (200g)	600	20	5
Processed Cheese	1 slice (21g)	350	9	2
Processed Meat Pizzas	1 slice (120g)	680	20	4
Regular Soda	1 can (355ml)	10	0	39
Store-Bought Cookies	4 cookies (56g)	210	12	24
Sweetened Almond Milk	1 cup (240ml)	150	3.5	16
Sweetened Condensed Milk	1 oz (28g)	35	3	22
White Bread	1 slice (28g)	150	1	2
White Pasta	1 cup (140g)	5	1.5	2.5
White Rice	1 cup (158g)	0	0.4	0.1

PHASES OF THE RICE DIET

Phase 1

Detoxification and Initial Weight Loss

The Rice Diet, initially developed for medical purposes, has evolved into a popular weight loss and detoxification regimen. Phase 1 of this diet is pivotal, setting the foundation for the transformative journey ahead. This initial phase, characterized by a strict eating plan, focuses on detoxifying the body and kickstarting the weight loss process. Participants often observe significant changes during this period, both physically and mentally, as they adapt to a new way of nourishing their bodies.

Diet Composition

At the heart of Phase 1 is the diet's composition, which is meticulously designed to promote health while minimizing calories. The primary component, as the name suggests, is rice. White or brown rice serves as the staple, providing a source of complex carbohydrates that release energy slowly, ensuring sustained satiety and energy levels throughout the day. Accompanying rice are various fruits and vegetables, chosen for their nutrient density and low-calorie profiles. These plant-based foods supply essential vitamins, minerals, and fiber, supporting digestive health and enhancing the body's detoxification processes.

Participants are encouraged to consume these foods in their natural, unprocessed forms to maximize nutrient intake and minimize exposure to added sugars and unhealthy fats. The diet strictly limits protein sources in this phase, focusing on plant-based proteins to reduce the strain on the digestive system and kidneys. Daily fluid intake is emphasized, with a recommendation for ample water consumption to aid in flushing toxins from the body.

Expected Benefits

The benefits of Phase 1 extend beyond mere weight loss. Participants often report improved energy levels, better digestion, and a noticeable reduction in bloating and inflammation. The high fiber content of the diet aids in regular bowel movements, crucial for detoxifying the body. Additionally, this phase can help recalibrate taste preferences, reducing cravings for sugary and fatty foods and fostering a new appreciation for the natural flavors of whole foods.

Weight loss during this phase can be quite significant, with many experiencing a rapid drop in pounds. This is partly due to the reduction in calorie intake and the body's initial response to a cleaner diet. The detoxification process also contributes to a better metabolic rate, preparing the body for continued weight loss in the subsequent phases.

Challenges and How to Overcome Them

Adapting to Phase 1 of the rice diet can be challenging. Participants might struggle with cravings, especially for those accustomed to high-sugar, high-fat diets. To combat this, it's recommended to keep a variety of allowed foods on hand, ensuring meals are satisfying and cravings for disallowed foods are minimized. Drinking plenty of water and herbal teas can also help manage hunger and cravings.

Social situations may pose another challenge, as dining out or attending events can make adherence to the diet difficult. Planning ahead by reviewing restaurant menus or eating a small, diet-compliant meal before events can help maintain commitment without feeling socially isolated.

Phase 2

Transition and Continued Weight Loss

As participants move into Phase 2 of the Rice Diet, the focus shifts from detoxification and initial weight loss to sustainable, continued weight loss and lifestyle integration. This phase is designed to build upon the foundation laid in Phase 1, introducing more variety into the diet while maintaining a calorie deficit conducive to weight loss. The goal is to transition into a more manageable and less restrictive diet that participants can adhere to for the long term.

Diet Adjustments and Diversification

Phase 2 allows for a broader range of foods, including the reintroduction of lean proteins and a wider variety of fruits, vegetables, and whole grains. This phase emphasizes the importance of a balanced diet that includes all macronutrients: carbohydrates, proteins, and fats, in a healthier form. The introduction of lean protein sources, such as fish, poultry, and plant-based proteins, supports muscle maintenance and overall health. Whole grains continue to be a staple, but now with greater variety, including quinoa, barley, and oats, providing essential nutrients and keeping hunger at bay.

Participants are encouraged to experiment with new recipes and flavors, incorporating diverse ingredients to keep meals interesting and nutritionally balanced. Portion control remains crucial, as does the careful monitoring of calorie intake to ensure continued weight loss. The flexibility in food choices helps address nutritional needs more effectively, making the diet easier to follow and more enjoyable.

Physical Activity Integration

Exercise becomes more integral in Phase 2, working synergistically with dietary adjustments to promote weight loss and enhance overall fitness. Participants are encouraged to engage in regular physical activity tailored to their fitness level and preferences. This might include aerobic exercises, strength training, and flexibility exercises. The aim is to find a sustainable and enjoyable routine that complements the dietary aspect of the rice diet.

Adjusting caloric intake to accommodate increased activity levels is important to ensure the body receives enough fuel for exercise without compromising weight loss goals. Regular physical activity not only aids in weight loss but also improves cardiovascular health, boosts mood, and increases energy levels.

Monitoring Progress and Adjustments

Ongoing monitoring of weight and health markers is vital in Phase 2. Regular check-ins help participants gauge their progress and make necessary adjustments to their diet and exercise routines. Dealing with weight loss plateaus is a common challenge; strategically altering calorie intake or exercise patterns can help overcome these stalls.

Feedback from the body, in terms of energy levels, hunger, and overall well-being, provides invaluable insight into how well the diet is working for an individual. Adjustments may be needed to tailor the diet more closely to individual needs, ensuring continued success.

Psychological Aspects and Motivation

Maintaining motivation through Phase 2 is crucial. The novelty of the diet may wear off, and the reality of long-term lifestyle changes can become daunting. It's important to celebrate small victories and set achievable, incremental goals to stay motivated. Finding a community of fellow dieters or a diet buddy can provide essential support, making the journey more enjoyable and less isolating. Sharing experiences, challenges, and successes helps keep motivation high and makes the diet a more sustainable and rewarding part of one's life.

Phase 3

Maintenance

Entering Phase 3 of the Rice Diet marks a significant transition from active weight loss to long-term maintenance. This phase is about integrating the principles learned during the initial stages into a sustainable lifestyle. The focus shifts to maintaining the weight loss achieved, preventing weight regain, and promoting overall health and well-being. It's a phase where flexibility and balance become key, allowing for a broader range of food choices while continuing to prioritize healthful eating habits.

Lifestyle Integration

The core of Phase 3 lies in making the Rice Diet a sustainable part of everyday life. This means adopting a balanced approach to eating that can be maintained indefinitely. Participants are encouraged to continue focusing on whole, nutrient-dense foods while allowing for occasional indulgences. The diet should be flexible enough to accommodate social events, travel, and special occasions without leading to weight regain.

Incorporating a wider variety of foods is important for nutritional balance and to prevent dietary boredom. Participants should aim to maintain a healthy balance of carbohydrates, proteins, and fats, focusing on the quality of these macronutrients. Whole grains, lean proteins, healthy fats, and a wide array of fruits and vegetables should form the basis of the diet.

Portion control remains crucial, as does listening to the body's hunger and fullness cues. Mindful eating practices can help maintain this balance, ensuring that food choices and portion sizes support weight maintenance and health goals.

Advanced Physical Activity

Physical activity in Phase 3 should be about maintaining fitness, building strength, and enhancing overall health. Participants are encouraged to diversify their exercise routines, incorporating activities that improve strength, flexibility, and cardiovascular health. Finding activities that are enjoyable and fit into one's lifestyle is key to long-term adherence.

Regular exercise not only helps in maintaining weight loss but also contributes to physical well-being, mental health, and a positive outlook on life. It's important to adjust exercise routines as needed to fit changing schedules, interests, and fitness levels, ensuring that physical activity remains a regular and enjoyable part of life.

Long-term Monitoring and Adjustments

Ongoing monitoring of weight and health indicators is essential in Phase 3. Regular check-ups with healthcare providers, along with self-monitoring of weight and dietary habits, help identify any issues early. Adjustments to the diet or exercise routine may be necessary in response to life changes, aging, or evolving health needs.

Recognizing signs of weight regain promptly and adjusting habits accordingly can help prevent backsliding. It's important to approach maintenance with flexibility, making changes as needed to sustain the achievements of the earlier phases.

Psychological and Social Considerations

Maintaining a positive mindset and motivation over the long term can be challenging. Setting new health and fitness goals, celebrating milestones, and engaging in activities that promote well-being can all help sustain motivation. Navigating social situations, dining out, and holidays requires planning and strategies to make healthful choices while enjoying life's pleasures.

Building a support network of friends, family, or others who share similar goals can provide encouragement, advice, and accountability. This network can be invaluable in navigating the challenges of maintaining long-term health and wellness.

IMPLEMENTING THE RICE DIET

Planning and Preparing Meals

Implementing the Rice Diet successfully hinges on meticulous planning and meal preparation. This high-complex carbohydrate, low-fat, and low-sodium diet requires a strategic approach to ensure nutritional adequacy and variety, making meal planning and prep paramount to adherence and enjoyment.

Weekly Meal Planning Guide

Understanding the Basics of the Rice Diet

The Rice Diet, originally developed for the treatment of hypertension and kidney disease, emphasizes whole grains, fruits, vegetables, and lean proteins. Understanding these foundational elements is crucial for creating a compliant meal plan.

Creating a Varied Meal Plan

Diversity in your meal plan ensures a range of nutrients and keeps the diet interesting. Include a variety of whole grains, not just rice, and rotate through different fruits, vegetables, and lean protein sources each week.

Shopping List Creation and Grocery Shopping Tips

A detailed shopping list aligned with your meal plan prevents impulse buys and ensures you have everything needed for the week. Focus on whole foods and avoid processed items to stay true to the diet's principles.

Meal Preparation Strategies

Batch Cooking and Portion Control

Preparing meals in large batches saves time and guarantees you have Rice Diet-friendly meals on hand. Portion out meals into individual containers for convenience and to avoid overeating.

Storage and Reheating Tips

Proper storage extends the freshness and flavor of your meals. Use airtight containers and follow safe reheating practices to maintain the nutritional integrity of your food.

Incorporating Diversity and Enjoyment

Experimenting with Spices and Herbs

Spices and herbs add flavor without the need for salt or fat, making meals more enjoyable and varied.

Finding Rice Diet-Friendly Recipes

Seek out or create recipes that fit within the Rice Diet parameters. Online communities and cookbooks dedicated to healthy eating can be valuable resources.

Overcoming Common Challenges

Meal planning and preparation can be time-consuming and monotonous. Overcoming these challenges involves setting aside dedicated time for meal prep, involving family members in the process, and constantly seeking new recipes to keep things interesting.

Managing Hunger and Cravings

Transitioning to the Rice Diet can be challenging, especially when it comes to managing hunger and cravings. The diet's high-complex carbohydrate focus is designed to promote satiety and support weight management, but understanding how to effectively manage hunger and cravings is key to long-term adherence and success. This section delves into strategies for distinguishing between hunger and cravings, satisfying hunger with Rice Diet-compliant foods, and coping with cravings in healthy, sustainable ways.

Identifying True Hunger

True hunger is your body's physiological need for food, characterized by physical cues such as a growling stomach, low energy levels, and the ability to eat almost any food. It's important to recognize these signals and differentiate them from cravings, which are often driven by emotional needs, stress, or habit rather than physical hunger.

The Role of Mindful Eating

Mindful eating is a powerful tool in distinguishing between hunger and cravings. It involves paying full attention to the experience of eating and drinking, both inside and outside the body. By eating slowly and without distraction, you can better recognize your body's hunger and satiety signals, making it easier to eat according to your physical needs rather than emotional impulses.

Satisfying Foods within the Rice Diet

The Rice Diet is inherently satiating due to its emphasis on complex carbohydrates, fiber-rich fruits and vegetables, and lean proteins. These foods not only help to stabilize blood sugar levels but also promote a feeling of fullness. To manage hunger effectively:

- Prioritize whole grains like brown rice, quinoa, and barley, which are slowly digested and provide steady energy.

- Incorporate a variety of vegetables and fruits into each meal to add bulk and fiber, enhancing satiety without significantly increasing calorie intake.

- Include a source of lean protein with meals and snacks to help maintain muscle mass and promote fullness.

Importance of Hydration

Thirst is often mistaken for hunger. Staying well-hydrated can help prevent this confusion and aid in hunger management. Drinking water before meals can also contribute to a feeling of fullness, reducing the likelihood of overeating.

Timing Meals and Snacks Effectively

Regularly spaced meals and snacks can prevent extreme hunger, making it easier to make healthful choices and portions. Aim for a balance of carbohydrates, protein, and healthy fats at each meal to maximize satiety and energy levels throughout the day.

Healthy Alternatives for Common Cravings

Cravings for specific tastes or textures can often be satisfied with healthier alternatives. For sweet cravings, fresh fruit or a small serving of dried fruit can be satisfying. For salty or crunchy cravings, try air-popped popcorn without added butter or salt. Look for Rice Diet-friendly recipes that mimic the flavors of your favorite treats in a healthier way.

Psychological Techniques to Combat Cravings

Understanding the emotional or situational triggers of your cravings can help you address them more effectively. Techniques such as distraction (engaging in a different activity), delay (waiting out the craving), and determination (reminding yourself of your dietary goals) can be effective strategies. Additionally, practicing stress-reduction techniques such as meditation, deep breathing, or gentle exercise can help manage the emotional drivers behind cravings.

Adapting to the Rice Diet is not just about making short-term changes; it's about developing a new relationship with food. Over time, the diet's high-fiber, low-fat approach can recalibrate your hunger cues and taste preferences, making it easier to manage hunger and cravings sustainably. Regular reflection on your eating habits, continued experimentation with new foods and recipes, and seeking support from a community or a healthcare professional can all contribute to lasting success on the Rice Diet.

Managing hunger and cravings is a critical aspect of the Rice Diet that requires both understanding and strategy. By learning to differentiate between hunger and cravings, incorporating satisfying foods into your diet, and developing techniques to cope with cravings, you can navigate the challenges of dietary change with confidence. The key is to approach these challenges with patience and flexibility, adapting strategies as you learn more about your body's needs and preferences. With time and practice, managing hunger and cravings can become a natural and rewarding part of your journey on the Rice Diet.

Dining Out and Social Events

Adhering to the Rice Diet doesn't mean you have to forgo dining out or attending social events. While these situations can present challenges, with a bit of planning and savvy, you can navigate them successfully without derailing your dietary goals. This guide will provide you with strategies to enjoy the social aspects of dining while staying true to the principles of the Rice Diet.

Tips for Dining Out

Choosing Rice Diet-Friendly Restaurants

Start by selecting restaurants that offer a variety of plant-based or whole food options. Many establishments now cater to health-conscious diners, making it easier to find dishes that fit within the Rice Diet parameters. Ethnic restaurants, such as Indian, Thai, or Japanese, often have a wealth of vegetarian dishes that emphasize rice, vegetables, and legumes.

What to Order from the Menu

Look for menu items that are steamed, grilled, or baked rather than fried. Opt for dishes that feature whole grains, vegetables, and lean proteins. Don't hesitate to ask for modifications to your order, such as dressing on the side or substituting a side dish to better align with your dietary needs. Restaurants are generally accommodating of such requests.

Communicating Dietary Needs with Restaurant Staff

Be clear but polite when explaining your dietary restrictions to your server. A simple explanation that you're following a low-fat, low-sodium diet for health reasons is usually enough. Most servers are willing to provide recommendations or communicate with the kitchen to ensure your needs are met.

Navigating Social Events

Planning Ahead for Social Gatherings

Before attending a social event, consider eating a small, Rice Diet-compliant meal or snack. This can help you avoid hunger and make it easier to resist temptations. Additionally, consider bringing a dish to share that fits within your dietary guidelines. This not only ensures there's something you can eat but also introduces others to your healthy lifestyle.

Healthy Snacking and Portion Control Tips

When faced with a buffet or snack table, fill your plate with vegetables, fruits, and whole grains first. These fiber-rich foods can help you feel full and satisfied, reducing the temptation to overindulge in less healthy options. Practice mindful eating by paying attention to your hunger cues and stopping when you're full.

How to Politely Decline Non-Compliant Foods

It's inevitable that you'll be offered foods that don't fit within your dietary plan. Politely declining with a simple "No, thank you" is usually sufficient. If pressed, you can explain that you're following a specific dietary plan for health reasons. Most hosts will understand and respect your dietary choices.

Enjoying Social Life While Maintaining Dietary Discipline

Maintaining the Rice Diet while engaging in social activities is about balance and flexibility. By planning ahead, making informed choices, and communicating your needs, you can fully participate in social life without compromising your dietary goals. Remember, the Rice Diet is not just about restrictions; it's a pathway to a healthier lifestyle that can still include the pleasure of dining out and socializing.

Navigating dining out and social events while on the Rice Diet requires awareness, preparation, and a willingness to advocate for your dietary needs. By employing the strategies outlined in this guide, you can enjoy a vibrant social life and delicious meals out, all while adhering to the diet's principles. The key is to approach these situations with confidence and a plan, ensuring that you can maintain your dietary discipline in a variety of settings. With these tools, the Rice Diet can seamlessly integrate into your lifestyle, allowing you to achieve your health goals without missing out on the joys of social dining.

Adjustments for Personal Preferences and Nutritional Needs

A one-size-fits-all approach rarely works in dietary planning, and the Rice Diet is no exception. Personal tastes, nutritional needs, and lifestyle factors play a significant role in the success of any diet plan. Adjusting the Rice Diet to accommodate these variables ensures not only adherence but also satisfaction and nutritional balance.

Tailoring the Diet to Personal Tastes

Exploring Alternative Grains

While rice is a staple of the diet, incorporating a variety of whole grains can enhance nutritional value and prevent monotony. Quinoa, barley, farro, and bulgur offer diverse textures and flavors, as well as additional nutrients. Experimenting with different grains keeps meals interesting and caters to personal taste preferences.

Incorporating Preferred Vegetables, Fruits, and Protein Sources

The Rice Diet is flexible enough to accommodate a wide range of vegetables, fruits, and lean proteins. Choose seasonal produce to ensure freshness and variety throughout the year. For proteins, consider plant-based options like lentils, beans, and tofu, or lean animal proteins if permitted. Tailoring these choices to your preferences supports dietary satisfaction and adherence.

Adjusting for Nutritional Needs

Modifications for Athletes or Those with High Energy Expenditures

Individuals with high physical activity levels may require adjustments to the Rice Diet to meet increased energy and nutritional demands. Incorporating a greater proportion of protein and complex carbohydrates can support energy needs and muscle recovery. It's essential to listen to your body and adjust portions and meal frequency accordingly.

Accommodating Dietary Restrictions and Allergies

For those with food allergies or specific dietary restrictions, the Rice Diet can be modified to ensure safety and nutritional adequacy. Substitute allergenic foods with safe alternatives that provide similar nutritional profiles. For example, if you're allergic to nuts, seeds can be a nutritious alternative for healthy fats.

Monitoring and Adjusting the Diet over Time

Tracking Progress and Nutritional Intake

Keeping a food diary can be helpful in monitoring adherence to the diet, understanding eating patterns, and identifying areas for adjustment. It also allows for tracking nutritional intake to ensure you're meeting your dietary needs.

When to Consider Adjustments and How to Make Them

If you find yourself feeling fatigued, experiencing digestive issues, or not meeting your health and weight goals, it may be time to adjust your diet. Consultation with a dietitian can provide personalized advice, ensuring your diet is balanced and meets your nutritional needs.

Consulting with Healthcare Professionals for Personalized Guidance While the Rice Diet has proven benefits, individual health conditions and nutritional requirements can necessitate professional guidance. A healthcare provider or dietitian can offer tailored advice, taking into account your health status, dietary preferences, and lifestyle factors. This personalized approach ensures the diet supports your overall health and well-being.

Adjusting the Rice Diet for personal preferences and nutritional needs is crucial for its long-term success and sustainability. By personalizing the diet, you can enjoy a variety of foods that cater to your tastes and meet your nutritional requirements, making it easier to adhere to and enjoy the benefits of the diet. Remember, the goal is not only weight management or health improvement but also to foster a positive relationship with food that can last a lifetime. Tailoring the diet to your individual needs and preferences is a key step in achieving this balance, ensuring that the Rice Diet becomes a feasible and enjoyable part of your lifestyle.

BREAKFAST RECIPES

Basic Brown Rice Porridge

Prep Time: 5 minutes

Cooking Time: 25 minutes

Serving Size: 1 bowl

Ingredients:

- 1 cup cooked brown rice
- 2 cups almond milk
- 1/2 teaspoon vanilla extract
- 1/4 teaspoon cinnamon
- 1 tablespoon maple syrup

Instructions:

1. In a medium saucepan, combine cooked brown rice and almond milk. Bring to a simmer over medium heat.
2. Add vanilla extract and cinnamon. Stir well.
3. Reduce heat to low and simmer, stirring occasionally, until it thickens to your liking, about 20 minutes.
4. Serve warm, drizzled with maple syrup.

Nutritional Information (per bowl):

- Calories: 220
- Protein: 4g
- Carbohydrates: 44g
- Dietary Fiber: 3g
- Fat: 3g

- Saturated Fat: 0g
- Sodium: 120mg
- Potassium: 150mg

Fruit Salad with Lemon Mint Dressing

Prep Time: 15 minutes

Cooking Time: 0 minutes

Serving Size: 1 cup

Ingredients:

- 1 cup mixed berries (strawberries, blueberries, raspberries)
- 1 medium banana, sliced
- 1 apple, diced
- Dressing:
- Juice of 1 lemon
- 1 tablespoon chopped fresh mint
- 1 teaspoon honey (optional)

Instructions:

1. In a large bowl, combine the mixed berries, banana, and apple.
2. In a small bowl, whisk together lemon juice, chopped mint, and honey if using.
3. Pour the dressing over the fruit and toss gently to combine.

Nutritional Information (per cup):

- Calories: 100
- Protein: 1g
- Carbohydrates: 25g
- Dietary Fiber: 4g

- Fat: 0g

- Saturated Fat: 0g

- Sodium: 5mg

- Potassium: 200mg

Rice Cakes with Avocado

Prep Time: 5 minutes

Cooking Time: 0 minutes

Serving Size: 2 rice cakes

Ingredients:

- 2 rice cakes

- 1 ripe avocado, mashed

- Salt and pepper to taste

- Chili flakes (optional)

Instructions:

1. Spread the mashed avocado evenly over the rice cakes.

2. Season with salt, pepper, and chili flakes if desired.

Nutritional Information (per serving):

- Calories: 200

- Protein: 3g

- Carbohydrates: 27g

- Dietary Fiber: 7g

- Fat: 10g

- Saturated Fat: 1.5g

- Sodium: 100mg

- Potassium: 500mg

Apple Cinnamon Rice Breakfast

Prep Time: 5 minutes

Cooking Time: 20 minutes

Serving Size: 1 bowl

Ingredients:

- 1 cup cooked brown rice

- 1 apple, diced

- 1/2 teaspoon cinnamon

- 1 cup almond milk

- 1 tablespoon raisins

- 1 tablespoon chopped walnuts

Instructions:

1. In a saucepan, combine brown rice, diced apple, cinnamon, and almond milk.

2. Cook over medium heat until the mixture is warm and the apple is tender, about 15 minutes.

3. Stir in raisins.

4. Serve topped with chopped walnuts.

Nutritional Information (per bowl):

- Calories: 300

- Protein: 5g

- Carbohydrates: 55g

- Dietary Fiber: 6g

- Fat: 8g

- Saturated Fat: 0.5g

- Sodium: 80mg

- Potassium: 350mg

Tropical Rice Smoothie

Prep Time: 5 minutes

Cooking Time: 0 minutes

Serving Size: 1 smoothie

Ingredients:

- 1/2 cup cooked white rice

- 1 cup coconut milk

- 1/2 banana

- 1/2 cup pineapple chunks

- 1 tablespoon honey (optional)

Instructions:

1. Combine all ingredients in a blender.

2. Blend until smooth.

Nutritional Information (per smoothie):

- Calories: 350

- Protein: 3g

- Carbohydrates: 60g

- Dietary Fiber: 2g

- Fat: 12g

- Saturated Fat: 10g

- Sodium: 50mg

- Potassium: 400mg

Peachy Rice Breakfast Bowl

Prep Time: 5 minutes

Cooking Time: 0 minutes (assuming rice is pre-cooked)

Serving Size: 1 bowl

Ingredients:

- 1 cup cooked brown rice
- 1 fresh peach, sliced
- 1/2 cup almond milk
- 1 tablespoon chia seeds
- 1/2 teaspoon vanilla extract
- 1 teaspoon honey (optional)

Instructions:

1. In a serving bowl, combine the cooked brown rice and almond milk.
2. Top with sliced peach and sprinkle with chia seeds.
3. Add vanilla extract and drizzle with honey if desired.

Nutritional Information (per bowl):

- Calories: 280
- Protein: 6g
- Carbohydrates: 55g
- Dietary Fiber: 8g
- Fat: 5g
- Saturated Fat: 0.5g
- Sodium: 80mg

- Potassium: 300mg

Savory Rice and Spinach Pancakes

Prep Time: 10 minutes

Cooking Time: 10 minutes

Serving Size: 2 pancakes

Ingredients:

- 1 cup cooked brown rice
- 1 cup fresh spinach, chopped
- 2 eggs, beaten
- 1/4 cup almond milk
- Salt and pepper to taste
- 1 tablespoon olive oil for cooking

Instructions:

1. In a bowl, mix together cooked brown rice, chopped spinach, beaten eggs, and almond milk. Season with salt and pepper.
2. Heat olive oil in a skillet over medium heat.
3. Pour half of the batter into the skillet to form a pancake.
4. Cook for about 5 minutes on each side or until golden brown. Repeat with the remaining batter.

Nutritional Information (per serving):

- Calories: 250
- Protein: 10g
- Carbohydrates: 30g
- Dietary Fiber: 4g
- Fat: 10g

- Saturated Fat: 2g

- Sodium: 200mg

- Potassium: 300mg

Rice and Berry Parfait

Prep Time: 10 minutes

Cooking Time: 0 minutes

Serving Size: 1 parfait

Ingredients:

- 1 cup cooked white rice, cooled

- 1/2 cup Greek yogurt

- 1/2 cup mixed berries (strawberries, blueberries, raspberries)

- 1 tablespoon honey (optional)

- A sprinkle of cinnamon (optional)

Instructions:

1. In a glass, layer half of the cooked rice, followed by a layer of Greek yogurt, and then a layer of mixed berries.

2. Repeat the layering process with the remaining ingredients.

3. Drizzle with honey and sprinkle with cinnamon if desired.

Nutritional Information (per parfait):

- Calories: 350

- Protein: 15g

- Carbohydrates: 65g

- Dietary Fiber: 4g

- Fat: 2g

- Saturated Fat: 1g

- Sodium: 70mg

- Potassium: 250mg

Rice and Nutmeg Porridge

Prep Time: 5 minutes

Cooking Time: 20 minutes

Serving Size: 1 bowl

Ingredients:

- 1 cup cooked brown rice

- 2 cups almond milk

- 1/4 teaspoon ground nutmeg

- 1 tablespoon maple syrup

- 1/4 cup raisins

Instructions:

1. In a medium saucepan, combine cooked brown rice, almond milk, and ground nutmeg. Bring to a simmer over medium heat.

2. Add raisins and maple syrup. Stir well.

3. Reduce heat to low and continue to simmer, stirring occasionally, until the mixture thickens, about 15-20 minutes.

Nutritional Information (per bowl):

- Calories: 300

- Protein: 5g

- Carbohydrates: 60g

- Dietary Fiber: 4g

- Fat: 4g

- Saturated Fat: 0g

- Sodium: 120mg

- Potassium: 300mg

Tropical Rice Pudding

Prep Time: 5 minutes

Cooking Time: 30 minutes

Serving Size: 1 bowl

Ingredients:

- 1 cup cooked white rice

- 2 cups coconut milk

- 1/4 cup sugar

- 1/2 cup diced pineapple

- 1/2 teaspoon vanilla extract

- Toasted coconut flakes for garnish

Instructions:

1. In a saucepan, combine cooked white rice, coconut milk, and sugar. Cook over medium heat, stirring occasionally, until the mixture thickens, about 20-30 minutes.

2. Remove from heat and stir in diced pineapple and vanilla extract.

3. Serve warm or chilled, garnished with toasted coconut flakes.

Nutritional Information (per bowl):

- Calories: 400

- Carbohydrates: 50g

- Dietary Fiber: 2g

- Fat: 20g
- Saturated Fat: 18g
- Sodium: 50mg
- Potassium: 200mg

LUNCH RECIPES

Rice and Bean Salad

Prep Time: 15 minutes

Cooking Time: 0 minutes (assuming rice and beans are pre-cooked)

Serving Size: 1 cup

Ingredients:

- 1 cup cooked brown rice
- 1 cup cooked black beans, rinsed and drained
- 1/2 cup diced red bell pepper
- 1/4 cup chopped cilantro
- 2 tablespoons lime juice
- 1 tablespoon olive oil
- Salt and pepper to taste

Instructions:

1. In a large bowl, combine brown rice, black beans, red bell pepper, and cilantro.
2. In a small bowl, whisk together lime juice, olive oil, salt, and pepper.
3. Pour the dressing over the rice mixture and toss to combine.

Nutritional Information (per cup):

- Calories: 220
- Protein: 8g
- Carbohydrates: 38g
- Dietary Fiber: 7g

- Fat: 5g

- Saturated Fat: 0.7g

- Sodium: 200mg

- Potassium: 400mg

Vegetable Stir-Fry over Brown Rice

Prep Time: 10 minutes

Cooking Time: 15 minutes

Serving Size: 1 plate

Ingredients:

- 1 cup cooked brown rice

- 2 cups mixed vegetables (broccoli, carrots, bell peppers, snap peas)

- 1 tablespoon soy sauce (low sodium)

- 1 teaspoon sesame oil

- 1 clove garlic, minced

- 1 teaspoon grated ginger

Instructions:

1. Heat sesame oil in a large skillet over medium heat. Add garlic and ginger, sautéing until fragrant.

2. Add mixed vegetables and stir-fry until tender-crisp, about 5-7 minutes.

3. Stir in soy sauce and cook for an additional minute.

4. Serve the vegetable mixture over cooked brown rice.

Nutritional Information (per plate):

- Calories: 320

- Protein: 8g

- Carbohydrates: 60g

- Dietary Fiber: 8g

- Fat: 5g

- Saturated Fat: 0.9g

- Sodium: 300mg

- Potassium: 500mg

Mushroom Rice Soup

Prep Time: 10 minutes

Cooking Time: 30 minutes

Serving Size: 1 bowl

Ingredients:

- 1 cup cooked brown rice

- 2 cups vegetable broth

- 1 cup sliced mushrooms

- 1/2 cup diced onions

- 1 clove garlic, minced

- 1 tablespoon olive oil

- Salt and pepper to taste

Instructions:

1. In a pot, heat olive oil over medium heat. Add onions and garlic, sautéing until translucent.

2. Add mushrooms and cook until they begin to soften.

3. Pour in vegetable broth and bring to a simmer.

4. Add cooked brown rice and season with salt and pepper. Simmer for 20 minutes.

Nutritional Information (per bowl):

- Calories: 200
- Protein: 5g
- Carbohydrates: 35g
- Dietary Fiber: 4g
- Fat: 5g
- Saturated Fat: 0.7g
- Sodium: 500mg
- Potassium: 300mg

Rice-Stuffed Bell Peppers

Prep Time: 20 minutes

Cooking Time: 30 minutes

Serving Size: 1 stuffed pepper

Ingredients:

- 4 bell peppers, tops removed and seeded
- 1 cup cooked brown rice
- 1/2 cup corn kernels
- 1/2 cup black beans, rinsed and drained
- 1/2 cup diced tomatoes
- 1 teaspoon cumin
- 1/2 teaspoon chili powder
- Salt and pepper to taste

Instructions:

1. Preheat oven to 375°F (190°C).

2. In a bowl, mix together brown rice, corn, black beans, diced tomatoes, cumin, chili powder, salt, and pepper.

3. Stuff each bell pepper with the rice mixture and place in a baking dish.

4. Cover with foil and bake for 30 minutes, or until peppers are tender.

Nutritional Information (per stuffed pepper):

- Calories: 150
- Protein: 5g
- Carbohydrates: 30g
- Dietary Fiber: 6g
- Fat: 1g
- Saturated Fat: 0g
- Sodium: 200mg
- Potassium: 500mg

Curried Rice Salad

Prep Time: 15 minutes

Cooking Time: 0 minutes (assuming rice is pre-cooked)

Serving Size: 1 cup

Ingredients:

- 1 cup cooked brown rice
- 1/2 cup diced cucumber
- 1/2 cup diced carrots
- 1/4 cup raisins
- 2 tablespoons chopped almonds
- 1 tablespoon olive oil
- 1 teaspoon curry powder
- Salt and pepper to taste

Instructions:

1. In a large bowl, mix the cooked brown rice with diced cucumber, carrots, raisins, and chopped almonds.
2. In a small bowl, whisk together olive oil, curry powder, salt, and pepper.
3. Pour the dressing over the rice mixture and toss to combine evenly.

Nutritional Information (per cup):

- Calories: 240
- Protein: 5g
- Carbohydrates: 45g
- Dietary Fiber: 5g

- Fat: 7g

- Saturated Fat: 1g

- Sodium: 200mg

- Potassium: 350mg

Rice and Lentil Salad

Prep Time: 15 minutes

Cooking Time: 0 minutes (assuming rice and lentils are pre-cooked)

Serving Size: 1 cup

Ingredients:

- 1/2 cup cooked brown rice

- 1/2 cup cooked lentils

- 1/2 cup diced tomatoes

- 1/4 cup chopped parsley

- 2 tablespoons lemon juice

- 1 tablespoon olive oil

- Salt and pepper to taste

Instructions:

1. In a large bowl, combine cooked brown rice, lentils, diced tomatoes, and chopped parsley.

2. In a small bowl, whisk together lemon juice, olive oil, salt, and pepper.

3. Pour the dressing over the salad and toss well to combine.

Nutritional Information (per cup):

- Calories: 220

- Protein: 9g

- Carbohydrates: 35g

- Dietary Fiber: 8g

- Fat: 5g

- Saturated Fat: 0.7g

- Sodium: 200mg

- Potassium: 400mg

Asian Rice and Cabbage Salad

Prep Time: 20 minutes

Cooking Time: 0 minutes

Serving Size: 1 cup

Ingredients:

- 1 cup cooked white rice, cooled

- 2 cups shredded cabbage (mix of red and green)

- 1/2 cup shredded carrots

- 1/4 cup sliced green onions

- Dressing:

- 2 tablespoons rice vinegar

- 1 tablespoon soy sauce (low sodium)

- 1 teaspoon sesame oil

- 1 teaspoon honey

- 1 clove garlic, minced

Instructions:

1. In a large bowl, combine cooled white rice, shredded cabbage, carrots, and green onions.

2. In a small bowl, whisk together rice vinegar, soy sauce, sesame oil, honey, and minced garlic to create the dressing.

3. Pour the dressing over the salad and toss well to coat.

Nutritional Information (per cup):

- Calories: 150

- Protein: 3g

- Carbohydrates: 30g

- Dietary Fiber: 3g

- Fat: 2g

- Saturated Fat: 0.3g

- Sodium: 200mg

- Potassium: 200mg

Mediterranean Rice Tabbouleh

Prep Time: 15 minutes

Cooking Time: 0 minutes (assuming rice is pre-cooked)

Serving Size: 1 cup

Ingredients:

- 1 cup cooked brown rice, cooled

- 1 cup chopped fresh parsley

- 1/2 cup chopped fresh mint

- 1/2 cup diced tomatoes

- 1/4 cup diced cucumber

- 2 tablespoons olive oil

- 2 tablespoons lemon juice

- Salt and pepper to taste

Instructions:

1. In a large bowl, combine cooled brown rice with chopped parsley, mint, diced tomatoes, and cucumber.

2. Drizzle with olive oil and lemon juice, then season with salt and pepper.

3. Toss well to combine and let sit for a few minutes to allow flavors to meld.

Nutritional Information (per cup):

- Calories: 180
- Protein: 4g
- Carbohydrates: 30g
- Dietary Fiber: 4g
- Fat: 6g
- Saturated Fat: 0.8g
- Sodium: 200mg
- Potassium: 250mg

Rice and Chickpea Stuffed Avocados

Prep Time: 10 minutes

Cooking Time: 0 minutes

Serving Size: 1 stuffed avocado (2 halves)

Ingredients:

- 1 ripe avocado, halved and pitted
- 1/2 cup cooked brown rice
- 1/2 cup cooked chickpeas, rinsed and drained
- 1 tablespoon chopped cilantro

- 2 tablespoons lime juice

- Salt and pepper to taste

Instructions:

1. In a bowl, mix together cooked brown rice, chickpeas, chopped cilantro, lime juice, salt, and pepper.

2. Scoop out some of the avocado flesh to create more space, if desired, and chop it to add to the filling.

3. Fill each avocado half with the rice and chickpea mixture.

Nutritional Information (per stuffed avocado):

- Calories: 320

- Protein: 7g

- Carbohydrates: 35g

- Dietary Fiber: 13g

- Fat: 18g

- Saturated Fat: 2.5g

- Sodium: 200mg

- Potassium: 800mg

Cold Rice and Pea Soup

Prep Time: 10 minutes

Cooking Time: 20 minutes (plus chilling time)

Serving Size: 1 bowl

Ingredients:

- 1 cup cooked white rice

- 2 cups vegetable broth

- 1 cup green peas (fresh or frozen)

- 1/4 cup chopped mint

- 1/2 cup almond milk

- Salt and pepper to taste

Instructions:

1. In a pot, bring vegetable broth to a simmer and add green peas. Cook until peas are tender, about 5 minutes.

2. Add cooked rice and chopped mint to the pot. Remove from heat and let cool.

3. Once cooled, blend the mixture until smooth, adding almond milk to achieve the desired consistency.

4. Chill the soup for at least 2 hours. Season with salt and pepper before serving.

Nutritional Information (per bowl):

- Calories: 180

- Protein: 6g

- Carbohydrates: 35g

- Dietary Fiber: 4g

- Fat: 2g

- Saturated Fat: 0g

- Sodium: 300mg

- Potassium: 250mg

DINNER RECIPES

Lentil and Rice Stew

Prep Time: 10 minutes

Cooking Time: 40 minutes

Serving Size: 1 bowl

Ingredients:

- 1/2 cup brown rice
- 1/2 cup green lentils
- 4 cups vegetable broth
- 1 carrot, diced
- 1 onion, diced
- 2 cloves garlic, minced
- 1 teaspoon cumin
- 1 teaspoon coriander
- Salt and pepper to taste

Instructions:

1. Rinse the lentils and rice under cold water.
2. In a large pot, sauté onion, garlic, and carrot with a splash of water until softened.
3. Add lentils, rice, vegetable broth, cumin, and coriander. Bring to a boil, then reduce heat to simmer.
4. Cover and cook for about 40 minutes, or until lentils and rice are tender.
5. Season with salt and pepper to taste.

Nutritional Information (per bowl):

- Calories: 250

- Protein: 12g

- Carbohydrates: 45g

- Dietary Fiber: 8g

- Fat: 1g

- Saturated Fat: 0g

- Sodium: 300mg

- Potassium: 400mg

Rice Primavera

Prep Time: 10 minutes

Cooking Time: 20 minutes

Serving Size: 1 cup

Ingredients:

- 1 cup cooked brown rice

- 1/2 cup chopped asparagus

- 1/2 cup peas

- 1/2 cup sliced carrots

- 1/4 cup diced bell pepper

- 1 tablespoon olive oil

- 1 clove garlic, minced

- 1 teaspoon lemon zest

- 2 tablespoons lemon juice

- Salt and pepper to taste

- 1 tablespoon chopped fresh parsley

Instructions:

1. Heat olive oil in a large skillet over medium heat. Add garlic and sauté until fragrant.
2. Add asparagus, peas, carrots, and bell pepper. Cook, stirring occasionally, until vegetables are tender but still crisp.
3. Stir in the cooked brown rice, lemon zest, and lemon juice. Cook for another 2-3 minutes to heat through.
4. Season with salt and pepper. Garnish with fresh parsley before serving.

Nutritional Information (per cup):

- Calories: 220
- Protein: 5g
- Carbohydrates: 40g
- Dietary Fiber: 5g
- Fat: 5g
- Saturated Fat: 0.7g
- Sodium: 200mg
- Potassium: 300mg

Cauliflower Rice Stir-Fry

Prep Time: 15 minutes

Cooking Time: 10 minutes

Serving Size: 1 cup

Ingredients:

- 2 cups cauliflower rice (grated cauliflower)
- 1 cup mixed vegetables (broccoli, carrots, bell peppers)
- 1 tablespoon soy sauce (low sodium)
- 1 teaspoon sesame oil
- 1 clove garlic, minced
- 1 teaspoon grated ginger

Instructions:

1. Heat sesame oil in a large skillet over medium heat. Add garlic and ginger, sautéing until fragrant.
2. Add mixed vegetables and stir-fry until tender-crisp.
3. Stir in cauliflower rice and soy sauce. Cook for 5-7 minutes, or until the cauliflower is tender.

Nutritional Information (per cup):

- Calories: 100
- Protein: 4g
- Carbohydrates: 15g
- Dietary Fiber: 4g
- Fat: 3g
- Saturated Fat: 0.5g
- Sodium: 300mg

- Potassium: 450mg

Tomato Basil Rice

Prep Time: 5 minutes

Cooking Time: 25 minutes

Serving Size: 1 cup

Ingredients:

- 1 cup cooked brown rice
- 1 cup diced tomatoes (fresh or canned)
- 1 tablespoon olive oil
- 2 cloves garlic, minced
- 1/4 cup fresh basil, chopped
- Salt and pepper to taste

Instructions:

1. Heat olive oil in a saucepan over medium heat. Add minced garlic and sauté until fragrant.
2. Stir in diced tomatoes and cook for about 5 minutes, until the tomatoes are softened.
3. Add the cooked brown rice to the saucepan, mixing well with the tomato mixture.
4. Cook for another 10 minutes on low heat, allowing the flavors to meld.
5. Remove from heat and stir in fresh basil. Season with salt and pepper to taste.

Nutritional Information (per cup):

- Calories: 210

- Protein: 4g

- Carbohydrates: 37g

- Dietary Fiber: 4g

- Fat: 5g

- Saturated Fat: 0.7g

- Sodium: 10mg

- Potassium: 250mg

Spinach and Lemon Rice

Prep Time: 5 minutes

Cooking Time: 20 minutes

Serving Size: 1 cup

Ingredients:

- 1 cup cooked brown rice

- 2 cups fresh spinach, chopped

- 1 tablespoon olive oil

- 2 tablespoons lemon juice

- 1 teaspoon lemon zest

- Salt and pepper to taste

Instructions:

1. In a large skillet, heat olive oil over medium heat. Add spinach and sauté until wilted.

2. Stir in the cooked brown rice, lemon juice, and lemon zest. Cook together for a few minutes until the rice is heated through.

3. Season with salt and pepper to taste.

Nutritional Information (per cup):

- Calories: 220
- Protein: 5g
- Carbohydrates: 38g
- Dietary Fiber: 4g
- Fat: 5g
- Saturated Fat: 0.7g
- Sodium: 200mg
- Potassium: 300mg

Rice and Lentil Salad

Prep Time: 10 minutes

Cooking Time: 20 minutes (if starting with uncooked rice and lentils)

Serving Size: 1 cup

Ingredients:

- 1/2 cup cooked brown rice
- 1/2 cup cooked green lentils
- 1/4 cup diced cucumber
- 1/4 cup diced tomato
- 1/4 cup chopped parsley
- 2 tablespoons lemon juice
- 1 tablespoon olive oil
- Salt and pepper to taste

Instructions:

1. In a large bowl, combine the cooked brown rice, cooked lentils, diced cucumber, diced tomato, and chopped parsley.
2. In a small bowl, whisk together lemon juice, olive oil, salt, and pepper to create the dressing.
3. Pour the dressing over the salad and toss to combine well.

Nutritional Information (per cup):

- Calories: 220
- Protein: 9g
- Carbohydrates: 38g
- Dietary Fiber: 9g
- Fat: 5g
- Saturated Fat: 0.7g
- Sodium: 200mg
- Potassium: 400mg

Asian Rice and Cabbage Salad

Prep Time: 15 minutes

Cooking Time: 0 minutes

Serving Size: 1 cup

Ingredients:

- 1 cup cooked white rice, cooled
- 2 cups shredded cabbage (a mix of red and green cabbage)
- 1/4 cup shredded carrots
- 1/4 cup sliced green onions
- Dressing:

- 2 tablespoons rice vinegar

- 1 tablespoon soy sauce (low sodium)

- 1 teaspoon sesame oil

- 1 teaspoon honey

- 1 clove garlic, minced

Instructions:

1. In a large bowl, combine cooled white rice, shredded cabbage, shredded carrots, and sliced green onions.

2. In a small bowl, whisk together rice vinegar, soy sauce, sesame oil, honey, and minced garlic to create the dressing.

3. Pour the dressing over the salad and toss well to coat.

Nutritional Information (per cup):

- Calories: 150

- Protein: 3g

- Carbohydrates: 30g

- Dietary Fiber: 3g

- Fat: 2g

- Saturated Fat: 0.3g

- Sodium: 200mg

- Potassium: 200mg

Mediterranean Rice Tabbouleh

Prep Time: 15 minutes

Cooking Time: 0 minutes

Serving Size: 1 cup

Ingredients:

- 1 cup cooked brown rice, cooled
- 1 cup chopped fresh parsley
- 1/2 cup chopped fresh mint
- 1/2 cup diced tomatoes
- 1/4 cup diced cucumber
- 2 tablespoons olive oil
- 2 tablespoons lemon juice
- Salt and pepper to taste

Instructions:

1. In a large bowl, combine cooled brown rice with chopped parsley, mint, diced tomatoes, and cucumber.
2. Drizzle with olive oil and lemon juice, then season with salt and pepper.
3. Toss well to combine and let sit for a few minutes to allow flavors to meld.

Nutritional Information (per cup):

- Calories: 180
- Protein: 4g
- Carbohydrates: 30g
- Dietary Fiber: 4g

- Fat: 6g
- Saturated Fat: 0.8g
- Sodium: 200mg
- Potassium: 250mg

Rice and Chickpea Stuffed Avocados

Prep Time: 10 minutes

Cooking Time: 0 minutes

Serving Size: 1 stuffed avocado (2 halves)

Ingredients:

- 1 ripe avocado, halved and pitted
- 1/2 cup cooked brown rice
- 1/2 cup cooked chickpeas, rinsed and drained
- 1 tablespoon chopped cilantro
- 2 tablespoons lime juice
- Salt and pepper to taste

Instructions:

1. In a bowl, mix together cooked brown rice, chickpeas, chopped cilantro, lime juice, salt, and pepper.
2. Scoop out some of the avocado flesh to create more space, if desired, and chop it to add to the filling.
3. 3Fill each avocado half with the rice and chickpea mixture.

Nutritional Information (per stuffed avocado):

- Calories: 320
- Protein: 7g
- Carbohydrates: 35g

- Dietary Fiber: 13g

- Fat: 18g

- Saturated Fat: 2.5g

- Sodium: 200mg

- Potassium: 800mg

Cold Rice and Pea Soup

Prep Time: 10 minutes

Cooking Time: 20 minutes (plus chilling time)

Serving Size: 1 bowl

Ingredients:

- 1 cup cooked white rice

- 2 cups vegetable broth

- 1 cup green peas (fresh or frozen)

- 1/4 cup chopped mint

- 1/2 cup almond milk

- Salt and pepper to taste

Instructions:

1. In a pot, bring vegetable broth to a simmer and add green peas. Cook until peas are tender, about 5 minutes.

2. Add cooked rice and chopped mint to the pot. Remove from heat and let cool.

3. Once cooled, blend the mixture until smooth, adding almond milk to achieve the desired consistency.

4. Chill the soup for at least 2 hours. Season with salt and pepper before serving.

Nutritional Information (per bowl):

- Calories: 180s
- Protein: 6g
- Carbohydrates: 35g
- Dietary Fiber: 4g
- Fat: 2g
- Saturated Fat: 0g
- Sodium: 300mg
- Potassium: 250mg

SNACKS AND SIDES

Asian Rice and Cabbage Salad

Prep Time: 15 minutes

Cooking Time: 0 minutes

Serving Size: 1 cup

Ingredients:

- 1 cup cooked white rice, cooled
- 2 cups shredded cabbage (mix of red and green for color)
- 1/4 cup shredded carrots
- 1/4 cup thinly sliced green onions
- 2 tablespoons rice vinegar
- 1 tablespoon soy sauce (low sodium)
- 1 teaspoon sesame oil
- 1 teaspoon honey (optional)
- 1 tablespoon sesame seeds

Instructions:

1. In a large bowl, combine the cooled white rice, shredded cabbage, carrots, and green onions.
2. In a small bowl, whisk together rice vinegar, soy sauce, sesame oil, and honey if using.
3. Pour the dressing over the rice and vegetables, tossing well to combine.
4. Sprinkle with sesame seeds before serving.

Nutritional Information (per cup):

- Calories: 150
- Protein: 3g
- Carbohydrates: 28g
- Dietary Fiber: 2g
- Fat: 3g
- Saturated Fat: 0.5g
- Sodium: 200mg
- Potassium: 150mg

Mediterranean Rice Tabbouleh

Prep Time: 15 minutes

Cooking Time: 0 minutes

Serving Size: 1 cup

Ingredients:

- 1 cup cooked brown rice, cooled
- 1 cup finely chopped fresh parsley
- 1/2 cup finely chopped fresh mint
- 1/2 cup diced tomatoes
- 1/4 cup diced cucumber
- 1/4 cup lemon juice
- 2 tablespoons olive oil
- Salt and pepper to taste

Instructions:

1. In a large bowl, mix the cooled brown rice with parsley, mint, tomatoes, and cucumber.

2. Dress with lemon juice and olive oil. Season with salt and pepper to taste.

3. Toss everything together until well combined.

Nutritional Information (per cup):

- Calories: 180
- Protein: 4g
- Carbohydrates: 27g
- Dietary Fiber: 3g
- Fat: 7g
- Saturated Fat: 1g
- Sodium: 10mg
- Potassium: 270mg

Rice and Chickpea Stuffed Avocados

Prep Time: 10 minutes

Cooking Time: 0 minutes

Serving Size: 2 halves

Ingredients:

- 1 ripe avocado, halved and pit removed
- 1/2 cup cooked brown rice
- 1/2 cup cooked chickpeas, rinsed and drained
- 1 tablespoon chopped cilantro
- 2 tablespoons lime juice
- Salt and pepper to taste

Instructions:

1. In a bowl, mix the cooked brown rice, chickpeas, and chopped cilantro.

2. Season the mixture with lime juice, salt, and pepper.

3. Spoon the rice and chickpea mixture into the avocado halves.

Nutritional Information (per 2 halves):

- Calories: 320

- Protein: 8g

- Carbohydrates: 38g

- Dietary Fiber: 14g

- Fat: 17g

- Saturated Fat: 2g

- Sodium: 200mg

- Potassium: 890mg

Cold Rice and Pea Soup

Prep Time: 10 minutes (plus cooling and chilling)

Cooking Time: 20 minutes

Serving Size: 1 bowl

Ingredients:

- 1 cup cooked white rice

- 2 cups vegetable broth

- 1 cup green peas (fresh or frozen)

- 1/4 cup fresh mint leaves

- 1/2 cup almond milk

- Salt and pepper to taste

Instructions:

1. In a saucepan, bring the vegetable broth to a boil and add the peas. Cook until tender.

2. Add the cooked rice and mint to the saucepan. Remove from heat and let cool slightly.

3. Puree the mixture in a blender until smooth, adding almond milk to reach the desired consistency.

4. Chill the soup for at least 2 hours. Season with salt and pepper before serving.

Nutritional Information (per bowl):

- Calories: 180
- Protein: 6g
- Carbohydrates: 36g
- Dietary Fiber: 4g
- Fat: 2g
- Saturated Fat: 0g
- Sodium: 300mg
- Potassium: 250mg

Cucumber Rice Vinegar Salad

Prep Time: 10 minutes

Cooking Time: 0 minutes

Serving Size: 1 cup

Ingredients:

- 2 large cucumbers, thinly sliced
- 1/4 cup rice vinegar
- 1 tablespoon honey (optional, or substitute with a sweetener of choice)
- 1 teaspoon sesame seeds
- Salt to taste

Instructions:

1. In a large bowl, combine the thinly sliced cucumbers with rice vinegar, honey (if using), and a pinch of salt. Mix well to ensure the cucumbers are evenly coated.
2. Let the mixture marinate for at least 10 minutes in the refrigerator to blend the flavors.
3. Before serving, sprinkle with sesame seeds for added texture and flavor.

Nutritional Information (per cup):

- Calories: 25
- Protein: 1g
- Carbohydrates: 6g (excluding optional honey)
- Dietary Fiber: 0.5g
- Fat: 0.5g

- Saturated Fat: 0g
- Sodium: 2mg
- Potassium: 184mg

Rice and Zucchini Fritters

Prep Time: 15 minutes

Cooking Time: 10 minutes

Serving Size: 2 fritters

Ingredients:

- 1 cup grated zucchini (water squeezed out)
- 1/2 cup cooked brown rice
- 1 egg, beaten
- 2 tablespoons whole wheat flour
- Salt and pepper to taste
- Olive oil for frying

Instructions:

1. Combine grated zucchini, cooked brown rice, beaten egg, whole wheat flour, salt, and pepper in a bowl. Stir until well mixed.
2. Heat a thin layer of olive oil in a skillet over medium heat.
3. Scoop portions of the mixture into the skillet, flattening them into fritter shapes. Cook for about 5 minutes on each side or until golden brown and crispy.

Nutritional Information (per 2 fritters):

- Calories: 200
- Protein: 6g

- Carbohydrates: 28g
- Dietary Fiber: 3g
- Fat: 7g
- Saturated Fat: 1.5g
- Sodium: 125mg
- Potassium: 270mg

Sweet Potato Rice Cakes

Prep Time: 20 minutes

Cooking Time: 30 minutes

Serving Size: 1 cake

Ingredients:

- 1 cup cooked and mashed sweet potato
- 1/2 cup cooked brown rice
- 1 egg (for binding)
- 1/4 teaspoon cinnamon
- 1 tablespoon maple syrup (optional)
- Olive oil for light brushing

Instructions:

1. Preheat your oven to 375°F (190°C). Line a baking sheet with parchment paper.

2. In a bowl, mix together mashed sweet potato, cooked brown rice, egg, cinnamon, and maple syrup if using.

3. Form the mixture into small cakes and place them on the prepared baking sheet. Brush the tops lightly with olive oil.

4. Bake for 15 minutes, then flip and bake for an additional 15 minutes or until the cakes are firm and lightly browned.

Nutritional Information (per cake):

- Calories: 90
- Protein: 2g
- Carbohydrates: 18g
- Dietary Fiber: 2g
- Fat: 1g
- Saturated Fat: 0g
- Sodium: 30mg
- Potassium: 160mg

Baked Rice Chips

Prep Time: 15 minutes (plus time to cook rice if not pre-cooked)

Cooking Time: 20 minutes

Serving Size: 10 chips

Ingredients:

- 1 cup cooked white rice, cooled
- 1 egg white
- Salt to taste
- Optional spices: paprika, garlic powder

Instructions:

1. Preheat oven to 350°F (175°C). Line a baking sheet with parchment paper.
2. Blend the cooked rice, egg white, and a pinch of salt (and any optional spices) in a food processor until smooth.

3. Spread the mixture thinly onto the prepared baking sheet. Bake for 10 minutes, then score into chip-sized pieces and bake for another 10 minutes or until crispy.

Nutritional Information (per 10 chips):

- Calories: 100
- Protein: 3g
- Carbohydrates: 22g
- Dietary Fiber: 0.5g
- Fat: 0.5g
- Saturated Fat: 0g
- Sodium: 75mg
- Potassium: 30mg

Rice and Kale Chips

Prep Time: 15 minutes

Cooking Time: 20 minutes

Serving Size: 1 cup

Ingredients:

- 1 cup cooked brown rice
- 2 cups kale, washed and torn into bite-size pieces
- 1 tablespoon olive oil
- Salt to taste

Instructions:

1. Preheat the oven to 300°F (150°C). Line a baking sheet with parchment paper.

2. In a large bowl, toss the kale pieces with olive oil and a pinch of salt until evenly coated.

3. Spread the kale on the prepared baking sheet in a single layer.

4. Sprinkle the cooked brown rice evenly over the kale.

5. Bake in the preheated oven for about 20 minutes, or until the kale is crispy and the rice is toasted.

Nutritional Information (per cup):

- Calories: 180
- Protein: 4g
- Carbohydrates: 27g
- Dietary Fiber: 2g
- Fat: 7g
- Saturated Fat: 1g
- Sodium: 200mg
- Potassium: 300mg

Rice and Lentil Salad

Prep Time: 15 minutes (plus cooking time if starting with uncooked rice and lentils)

Cooking Time: 0 minutes

Serving Size: 1 cup

Ingredients:

- 1/2 cup cooked brown rice
- 1/2 cup cooked green or brown lentils
- 1/4 cup diced red bell pepper
- 1/4 cup diced cucumber

- 1/4 cup halved cherry tomatoes
- 2 tablespoons finely chopped red onion
- 2 tablespoons chopped fresh parsley
- Dressing:
- 3 tablespoons olive oil
- 1 tablespoon lemon juice
- 1 teaspoon Dijon mustard
- 1 small garlic clove, minced
- Salt and pepper to taste

Instructions:

1. In a large bowl, combine the cooked brown rice and lentils.
2. Add the diced red bell pepper, cucumber, cherry tomatoes, red onion, and chopped parsley to the bowl.
3. In a small bowl or jar, whisk together the olive oil, lemon juice, Dijon mustard, minced garlic, salt, and pepper until well blended to create the dressing.
4. Pour the dressing over the salad and toss gently to ensure all the ingredients are evenly coated.
5. Let the salad sit for at least 10 minutes before serving to allow the flavors to meld. This salad can be served at room temperature or chilled, based on personal preference.

Nutritional Information (per cup):

- Calories: 220
- Protein: 8g
- Carbohydrates: 30g
- Dietary Fiber: 7g

- Saturated Fat: 1g
- Sodium: 100mg
- Potassium: 350mg

DESSERTS RECIPES

Fruit and Rice Pudding

Prep Time: 10 minutes

Cooking Time: 40 minutes

Serving Size: 1 cup

Ingredients:

- 1/2 cup uncooked brown rice
- 2 cups almond milk
- 1/4 teaspoon cinnamon
- 1/4 cup raisins
- 1 apple, peeled and diced
- 1 banana, sliced
- 1 tablespoon honey (optional)

Instructions:

1. Rinse the brown rice under cold water.
2. In a saucepan, combine the brown rice, almond milk, and cinnamon. Bring to a boil, then reduce heat to low, cover, and simmer for about 30 minutes, or until the rice is tender.
3. Stir in the raisins, diced apple, and slices of banana. Continue to cook for another 10 minutes, or until the fruit is soft.
4. Remove from heat and stir in honey if desired. Serve warm or chilled.

Nutritional Information (per cup):

- Calories: 220
- Protein: 4g

- Carbohydrates: 46g

- Dietary Fiber: 4g

- Fat: 2g

- Saturated Fat: 0g

- Sodium: 80mg

- Potassium: 300mg

Baked Apples with Rice and Cinnamon

Prep Time: 15 minutes

Cooking Time: 30 minutes

Serving Size: 1 apple

Ingredients:

- 4 large apples

- 1 cup cooked brown rice

- 2 tablespoons raisins

- 1 teaspoon cinnamon

- 1/4 cup chopped walnuts

- 1/4 cup honey

- 1/2 cup water

Instructions:

1. Preheat oven to 350°F (175°C).

2. Core the apples and scoop out some flesh to create a well. Chop the scooped-out apple flesh.

3. In a bowl, mix the cooked brown rice, chopped apple flesh, raisins, cinnamon, walnuts, and 2 tablespoons of honey.

4. Fill each apple with the rice mixture and place them in a baking dish.

5. Drizzle the remaining honey over the apples and add water to the bottom of the dish.

6. Bake for 30 minutes, or until apples are soft and the filling is bubbly.

Nutritional Information (per apple):

- Calories: 250
- Protein: 3g
- Carbohydrates: 53g
- Dietary Fiber: 6g
- Fat: 4g
- Saturated Fat: 0.5g
- Sodium: 10mg
- Potassium: 350mg

Rice and Carrot Halwa

Prep Time: 10 minutes

Cooking Time: 30 minutes

Serving Size: 1/2 cup

Ingredients:

- 1 cup grated carrots
- 1/2 cup cooked brown rice
- 2 cups almond milk
- 1/4 cup raisins
- 1/4 teaspoon cardamom powder

- 1 tablespoon ghee (or coconut oil for a vegan option)
- 2 tablespoons honey (adjust to taste)

Instructions:

1. In a large pan, heat the ghee (or coconut oil) over medium heat. Add the grated carrots and sauté for about 5 minutes, until they start to soften.
2. Add the cooked brown rice, almond milk, raisins, and cardamom powder to the pan. Stir well to combine.
3. Bring the mixture to a boil, then reduce the heat and simmer, stirring occasionally, until the milk is absorbed and the mixture thickens, about 20 minutes.
4. Stir in the honey and cook for another 5 minutes.
5. Serve warm or chilled, garnished with additional nuts or raisins if desired.

Nutritional Information (per 1/2 cup):

- Calories: 180
- Protein: 3g
- Carbohydrates: 30g
- Dietary Fiber: 3g
- Fat: 5g
- Saturated Fat: 3g (if using ghee)
- Sodium: 60mg
- Potassium: 200mg

Rice Flour Pancakes

Prep Time: 10 minutes

Cooking Time: 15 minutes

Serving Size: 2 pancakes

Ingredients:

- 1 cup rice flour
- 1 teaspoon baking powder
- 1/2 teaspoon salt
- 1 tablespoon honey or maple syrup
- 1 egg
- 1 cup almond milk
- 1 teaspoon vanilla extract
- Olive oil or coconut oil for cooking

Instructions:

1. In a mixing bowl, combine rice flour, baking powder, and salt.
2. In another bowl, whisk together the honey (or maple syrup), egg, almond milk, and vanilla extract.
3. Pour the wet ingredients into the dry ingredients and stir until just combined.
4. Heat a lightly oiled skillet over medium heat. Pour or scoop the batter onto the skillet, using approximately 1/4 cup for each pancake.
5. Cook until bubbles form and the edges are dry, about 2-3 minutes. Flip and cook until browned on the other side.

Nutritional Information (per 2 pancakes):

- Calories: 250
- Protein: 6g
- Carbohydrates: 45g
- Dietary Fiber: 2g
- Fat: 5g
- Saturated Fat: 1g
- Sodium: 600mg
- Potassium: 100mg

Banana Rice Cream

Prep Time: 5 minutes (plus chilling time if preferred)

Cooking Time: 0 minutes

Serving Size: 1/2 cup

Ingredients:

- 1 ripe banana
- 1/2 cup cooked white rice
- 1/4 cup coconut milk
- 1/2 teaspoon vanilla extract
- Pinch of cinnamon (optional)

Instructions:

1. In a blender, combine the ripe banana, cooked white rice, coconut milk, vanilla extract, and cinnamon if using.
2. Blend until smooth and creamy.
3. Serve immediately for a soft-serve texture or chill in the refrigerator for a firmer consistency.

Nutritional Information (per 1/2 cup):

- Calories: 150
- Protein: 2g
- Carbohydrates: 30g
- Dietary Fiber: 2g
- Fat: 3g
- Saturated Fat: 2g
- Sodium: 10mg
- Potassium: 220mg

Rice and Lentil Salad

Prep Time: 15 minutes (if starting with cooked rice and lentils)

Cooking Time: 0 minutes

Serving Size: 1 cup

Ingredients:

- 1/2 cup cooked brown rice
- 1/2 cup cooked green lentils
- 1/4 cup diced red bell pepper
- 1/4 cup diced cucumber
- 1/4 cup chopped fresh parsley
- Dressing:
- 2 tablespoons olive oil
- 1 tablespoon lemon juice
- 1 garlic clove, minced
- Salt and pepper to taste

Instructions:

1. In a large bowl, mix together the cooked brown rice, green lentils, red bell pepper, cucumber, and parsley.

2. In a small bowl, whisk together the olive oil, lemon juice, minced garlic, salt, and pepper to make the dressing.

3. Pour the dressing over the salad and toss until everything is evenly coated.

Nutritional Information (per cup):

- Calories: 220

- Protein: 9g

- Carbohydrates: 35g

- Dietary Fiber: 8g

- Fat: 7g

- Saturated Fat: 1g

- Sodium: 200mg

- Potassium: 400mg

Asian Rice and Cabbage Salad

Prep Time: 15 minutes

Cooking Time: 0 minutes

Serving Size: 1 cup

Ingredients:

- 1 cup cooked white rice, cooled

- 2 cups shredded cabbage

- 1/4 cup shredded carrots

- 1/4 cup thinly sliced green onions

- Dressing:
- 2 tablespoons soy sauce (low sodium)
- 2 tablespoons rice vinegar
- 1 teaspoon sesame oil
- 1 teaspoon honey
- 1 clove garlic, minced

Instructions:

1. In a large bowl, combine the cooled white rice, shredded cabbage, carrots, and green onions.
2. In a small bowl, whisk together the soy sauce, rice vinegar, sesame oil, honey, and minced garlic to create the dressing.
3. Pour the dressing over the salad and toss well to combine.

Nutritional Information (per cup):

- Calories: 150
- Protein: 3g
- Carbohydrates: 28g
- Dietary Fiber: 2g
- Fat: 3g
- Saturated Fat: 0.5g
- Sodium: 300mg
- Potassium: 150mg

Mediterranean Rice Tabbouleh

Prep Time: 20 minutes

Cooking Time: 0 minutes

Serving Size: 1 cup

Ingredients:

- 1 cup cooked brown rice, cooled
- 1 cup finely chopped fresh parsley
- 1/2 cup finely chopped fresh mint
- 1/2 cup diced tomatoes
- 1/4 cup diced cucumber
- 1/4 cup finely chopped red onion
- Dressing:
- 3 tablespoons olive oil
- 2 tablespoons lemon juice
- Salt and pepper to taste

Instructions:

1. In a large bowl, mix together the cooled brown rice, chopped parsley, mint, diced tomatoes, cucumber, and red onion.
2. In a small bowl, whisk together the olive oil and lemon juice, then season with salt and pepper.
3. Pour the dressing over the rice mixture and toss to combine thoroughly. Adjust seasoning if necessary.
4. Chill in the refrigerator for at least 30 minutes before serving to allow flavors to meld.

Nutritional Information (per cup):

- Calories: 200
- Protein: 4g
- Carbohydrates: 30g
- Dietary Fiber: 5g
- Fat: 8g
- Saturated Fat: 1g
- Sodium: 10mg
- Potassium: 300mg

Rice and Chickpea Stuffed Avocados

Prep Time: 15 minutes

Cooking Time: 0 minutes

Serving Size: 2 stuffed avocado halves

Ingredients:

- 1 large ripe avocado, halved and pit removed
- 1/2 cup cooked brown rice
- 1/2 cup cooked chickpeas, rinsed and drained
- 1/4 cup diced tomato
- 1/4 cup diced red onion
- 1 tablespoon chopped cilantro
- Dressing:
- 2 tablespoons lime juice
- 1 tablespoon olive oil
- Salt and pepper to taste

Instructions:

1. In a bowl, combine the cooked brown rice, chickpeas, diced tomato, red onion, and cilantro.
2. In a small bowl, whisk together lime juice, olive oil, salt, and pepper to create the dressing.
3. Drizzle the dressing over the rice and chickpea mixture, then toss to combine.
4. Carefully spoon the mixture into the avocado halves, filling them generously.
5. Serve immediately, garnished with additional cilantro if desired.

Nutritional Information (per 2 stuffed halves):

- Calories: 320
- Protein: 7g
- Carbohydrates: 35g
- Dietary Fiber: 15g
- Fat: 18g
- Saturated Fat: 2.5g

Cold Rice and Pea Soup

Prep Time: 10 minutes (plus chilling)

Cooking Time: 20 minutes

Serving Size: 1 bowl

Ingredients:

- 1 cup cooked white rice, cooled
- 2 cups vegetable broth
- 1 cup green peas (fresh or frozen)
- 1/4 cup fresh mint leaves, plus extra for garnish
- 1/2 cup almond milk or coconut milk
- Salt and pepper to taste
- Optional garnishes: a swirl of yogurt, olive oil, or additional fresh peas

Instructions:

1. In a medium saucepan, bring the vegetable broth to a boil. Add the green peas and cook until just tender, about 3-5 minutes for fresh peas or 5-7 minutes for frozen.

2. In a blender, combine the cooked peas (reserve some for garnish if desired), cooked rice, fresh mint leaves, and a portion of the cooking broth. Blend until smooth. Depending on your blender's size, you might need to do this in batches.

3. Transfer the blended mixture into a large bowl. Stir in the almond milk or coconut milk until well combined. Season with salt and pepper to taste.

4. Chill the soup in the refrigerator for at least 2 hours. It can also be left overnight if you prefer a colder soup.

5. Serve the soup cold, garnished with fresh mint leaves, a few whole peas, and a swirl of yogurt or a drizzle of olive oil if using.

Nutritional Information (per bowl):

- Calories: 150 (varies depending on the choice of milk and garnishes)

- Protein: 5g

- Carbohydrates: 28g

- Dietary Fiber: 4g

- Fat: 2g (varies with garnishes)

- Saturated Fat: 0.3g (varies with choice of milk and garnishes)

- Sodium: 300mg (can vary based on the vegetable broth and added salt)

- Potassium: 200mg

BEVERAGES RECIPES

Rice Milk Smoothie

Prep Time: 5 minutes

Cooking Time: 0 minutes

Serving Size: 2 cups

Ingredients:

- 1 cup rice milk
- 1 banana, sliced
- 1/2 cup mixed berries (strawberries, blueberries, raspberries)
- 1 tablespoon honey or maple syrup (optional)
- 1/2 teaspoon vanilla extract
- Ice cubes (optional)

Instructions:

1. In a blender, combine the rice milk, banana, mixed berries, honey or maple syrup (if using), and vanilla extract.
2. Blend until smooth. If the smoothie is too thick, you can add a little more rice milk to reach your desired consistency.
3. Add ice cubes to the blender if you prefer a colder smoothie and blend again until smooth.
4. Pour into glasses and serve immediately.

Nutritional Information (per cup):

- Calories: 150
- Protein: 2g
- Carbohydrates: 34g
- Dietary Fiber: 4g

- Fat: 1g

- Saturated Fat: 0g

- Sodium: 50mg

- Potassium: 300mg

- Calcium: 150mg

Golden Rice Tea

Prep Time: 5 minutes

Cooking Time: 10 minutes

Serving Size: 2 cups

Ingredients:

- 2 cups water

- 1 tablespoon green tea leaves

- 1/4 cup uncooked rice

- Honey or sugar to taste (optional)

- A slice of lemon for garnish (optional)

Instructions:

1. In a small pan, dry roast the rice over medium heat until golden brown, stirring frequently to prevent burning. Remove from heat and let cool.

2. Bring water to a boil in a kettle or pot.

3. Add the toasted rice and green tea leaves to the boiling water. Reduce heat and simmer for about 5 minutes.

4. Strain the tea into cups, discarding the rice and tea leaves.

5. Sweeten with honey or sugar if desired and garnish with a slice of lemon.

Nutritional Information (per cup):

- Calories: 10 (without sweeteners)
- Protein: 0g
- Carbohydrates: 2g
- Dietary Fiber: 0g
- Fat: 0g
- Saturated Fat: 0g
- Sodium: 0mg
- Potassium: 20mg

Rice Water with Lemon and Mint

Prep Time: 5 minutes (plus time for rice water to cool)

Cooking Time: 30 minutes

Serving Size: 4 cups

Ingredients:

- 1/2 cup uncooked rice
- 4 cups water
- 1 lemon, juice, and zest
- A handful of fresh mint leaves
- Honey or sugar to taste (optional)

Instructions:

1. Rinse the rice thoroughly under cold running water.

2. In a pot, combine the rinsed rice and water. Bring to a boil, then reduce heat and simmer for 30 minutes.

3. Strain the rice, reserving the water. Allow the rice water to cool to room temperature.

4. Once cooled, add the lemon juice and zest, and mint leaves to the rice water. Stir well.

5. Sweeten with honey or sugar if desired. Refrigerate until chilled.

6. Serve cold, garnished with extra mint leaves and lemon slices.

Nutritional Information (per cup):

- Calories: 20 (without sweeteners)
- Protein: 0g
- Carbohydrates: 5g
- Dietary Fiber: 0g
- Fat: 0g
- Saturated Fat: 0g
- Sodium: 10mg
- Potassium: 50mg

Cucumber Rice Water

Prep Time: 10 minutes (plus time for rice water to cool)

Cooking Time: 30 minutes

Serving Size: 4 cups

Ingredients:

- 1/2 cup uncooked rice
- 4 cups water
- 1 medium cucumber, thinly sliced
- Honey or sugar to taste (optional)
- A few sprigs of fresh dill for garnish (optional)

Instructions:

1. Rinse the rice thoroughly under cold water.
2. In a pot, bring the rice and water to a boil, then simmer for 30 minutes.
3. Strain the rice, keeping the water. Allow it to cool.
4. Add the cucumber slices to the cooled rice water. Refrigerate until chilled.
5. Sweeten with honey or sugar if desired. Serve cold, garnished with fresh dill.

Nutritional Information (per cup):

- Calories: 20 (without sweeteners)
- Protein: 0g
- Carbohydrates: 5g
- Dietary Fiber: 0.5g
- Fat: 0g
- Saturated Fat: 0g
- Sodium: 10mg
- Potassium: 75mg

Herbal Rice Tea

Prep Time: 5 minutes

Cooking Time: 10 minutes

Serving Size: 2 cups

Ingredients:

- 2 cups water
- 1/4 cup uncooked rice
- 1 teaspoon chamomile flowers
- 1 teaspoon mint leaves
- 1 teaspoon lavender flowers
- Honey or sugar to taste (optional)

Instructions:

1. In a small pan, dry roast the rice over medium heat until golden brown, stirring frequently to prevent burning. Remove from heat and let cool.
2. Bring water to a boil in a kettle or pot.
3. Add the toasted rice, chamomile flowers, mint leaves, and lavender flowers to the boiling water. Reduce heat and simmer for about 5 minutes.
4. Strain the tea into cups, discarding the rice and herbs.
5. Sweeten with honey or sugar if desired.

Nutritional Information (per cup):

- Calories: 15 (without sweeteners)
- Protein: 0g
- Carbohydrates: 3g

- Dietary Fiber: 0g

- Fat: 0g

- Saturated Fat: 0g

- Sodium: 0mg

- Potassium: 25mg

Rice and Lentil Salad

Prep Time: 10 minutes

Cooking Time: 20 minutes

Serving Size: 4 servings

Ingredients:

- 1 cup cooked brown rice

- 1 cup cooked green lentils

- 1/2 cup diced tomatoes

- 1/2 cup diced cucumber

- 1/4 cup finely chopped red onion

- 2 tablespoons olive oil

- 1 tablespoon lemon juice

- Salt and pepper to taste

- A handful of fresh parsley, chopped

Instructions:

1. In a large bowl, mix together the cooked brown rice and green lentils.

2. Add the diced tomatoes, cucumber, and red onion to the bowl.

3. In a small bowl, whisk together the olive oil and lemon juice. Pour this dressing over the salad and toss to combine.

4. Season with salt and pepper to taste. Garnish with chopped parsley.

5. Serve chilled or at room temperature.

Nutritional Information (per serving):

- Calories: 250
- Protein: 10g
- Carbohydrates: 38g
- Dietary Fiber: 8g
- Fat: 7g
- Saturated Fat: 1g
- Sodium: 30mg
- Potassium: 450mg

Asian Rice and Cabbage Salad

Prep Time: 15 minutes

Cooking Time: 0 minutes

Serving Size: 4 servings

Ingredients:

- 2 cups cooked jasmine rice, cooled
- 2 cups shredded purple cabbage
- 1 cup shredded carrots
- 1/2 cup thinly sliced red bell pepper
- 1/4 cup chopped green onions
- 1/4 cup chopped cilantro
- For the dressing:
- 2 tablespoons soy sauce

- 1 tablespoon rice vinegar
- 1 tablespoon sesame oil
- 1 teaspoon honey or sugar
- 1 garlic clove, minced
- 1 teaspoon grated ginger

Instructions:

1. In a large bowl, combine the cooked jasmine rice, shredded purple cabbage, carrots, red bell pepper, green onions, and cilantro.
2. In a small bowl, whisk together the soy sauce, rice vinegar, sesame oil, honey or sugar, minced garlic, and grated ginger to create the dressing.
3. Pour the dressing over the salad and toss until everything is well coated.
4. Let the salad sit for about 10 minutes before serving to allow the flavors to meld.

Nutritional Information (per serving):

- Calories: 220
- Protein: 4g
- Carbohydrates: 42g
- Dietary Fiber: 3g
- Fat: 5g
- Saturated Fat: 0.5g
- Sodium: 430mg
- Potassium: 300mg

Mediterranean Rice Tabbouleh

Prep Time: 15 minutes

Cooking Time: 0 minutes

Serving Size: 6 servings

Ingredients:

- 2 cups cooked brown rice, cooled
- 1 cup finely chopped fresh parsley
- 1/2 cup finely chopped fresh mint
- 1 cup diced tomatoes
- 1/2 cup diced cucumber
- 1/4 cup finely chopped red onion
- 3 tablespoons olive oil
- 2 tablespoons lemon juice
- Salt and pepper to taste

Instructions:

1. In a large bowl, combine the cooked brown rice, chopped parsley, mint, diced tomatoes, cucumber, and red onion.
2. Drizzle the olive oil and lemon juice over the salad. Toss well to combine.
3. Season with salt and pepper according to taste.
4. Refrigerate for at least 30 minutes before serving to allow the flavors to blend.

Nutritional Information (per serving):

- Calories: 180
- Protein: 3g

- Carbohydrates: 30g

- Dietary Fiber: 3g

- Fat: 6g

- Saturated Fat: 1g

- Sodium: 20mg

- Potassium: 250mg

Rice and Chickpea Stuffed Avocados

Prep Time: 20 minutes

Cooking Time: 0 minutes

Serving Size: 4 halves

Ingredients:

- 2 ripe avocados, halved and pitted

- 1 cup cooked brown rice

- 1/2 cup cooked chickpeas

- 1/4 cup diced tomatoes

- 1/4 cup diced red onion

- 2 tablespoons chopped cilantro

- Juice of 1 lime

- Salt and pepper to taste

- Optional: chili flakes for garnish

Instructions:

1. Scoop out a bit of the avocado flesh to create more space for the filling, leaving a border around the edges.

2. In a bowl, mix together the cooked brown rice, chickpeas, diced tomatoes, red onion, and chopped cilantro.

3. Squeeze lime juice over the mixture, and season with salt and pepper. Stir well to combine.

4. Spoon the rice and chickpea mixture into the avocado halves.

5. Garnish with chili flakes if desired. Serve immediately.

Nutritional Information (per half):

- Calories: 250

- Protein: 5g

- Carbohydrates: 27g

- Dietary Fiber: 10g

- Fat: 15g

- Saturated Fat: 2g

- Sodium: 30mg

- Potassium: 700mg

Cold Rice and Pea Soup

Prep Time: 10 minutes (plus chilling)

Cooking Time: 20 minutes

Serving Size: 4 servings

Ingredients:

- 1 cup cooked white rice

- 2 cups vegetable broth

- 1 cup fresh or frozen peas

- 1/2 cup chopped onion

- 1 garlic clove, minced

- 1 tablespoon olive oil

- Salt and pepper to taste

- Fresh mint leaves for garnish

Instructions:

1. In a saucepan, heat the olive oil over medium heat. Add the chopped onion and minced garlic, sautéing until soft and translucent.
2. Add the peas and vegetable broth to the saucepan. Bring to a boil, then reduce heat and simmer for 10 minutes.
3. Stir in the cooked rice and cook for another 5 minutes. Season with salt and pepper.
4. Remove from heat and let cool. Once cooled, blend the soup until smooth using a blender or immersion blender.
5. Chill the soup in the refrigerator for at least 2 hours before serving.
6. Serve cold, garnished with fresh mint leaves.

Nutritional Information (per serving):

- Calories: 180
- Protein: 4g
- Carbohydrates: 30g
- Dietary Fiber: 3g
- Fat: 5g
- Saturated Fat: 0.5g
- Sodium: 250mg
- Potassium: 150mg

21-DAY MEAL PLAN

Day 1

- Breakfast: Basic Brown Rice Porridge
- Lunch: Rice and Bean Salad
- Dinner: Lentil and Rice Stew
- Snacks: Sweet Potato Rice Cakes
- Dessert: Fruit and Rice Pudding
- Beverage: Rice Milk Smoothie

Day 2

- Breakfast: Fruit Salad with Lemon Mint Dressing
- Lunch: Vegetable Stir-Fry over Brown Rice
- Dinner: Tomato Basil Rice
- Snacks: Rice and Zucchini Fritters
- Dessert: Baked Apples with Rice and Cinnamon
- Beverage: Golden Rice Tea

Day 3

- Breakfast: Rice Cakes with Avocado
- Lunch: Mushroom Rice Soup
- Dinner: Cauliflower Rice Stir-Fry
- Snacks: Baked Rice Chips
- Dessert: Rice and Carrot Halwa
- Beverage: Rice Water with Lemon and Mint

Day 4

- Breakfast: Apple Cinnamon Rice Breakfast
- Lunch: Rice-Stuffed Bell Peppers
- Dinner: Spinach and Lemon Rice
- Snacks: Rice and Kale Chips
- Dessert: Rice Flour Pancakes
- Beverage: Cucumber Rice Water

Day 5

- Breakfast: Tropical Rice Smoothie
- Lunch: Curried Rice Salad
- Dinner: Rice Primavera
- Snacks: Cucumber Rice Vinegar Salad
- Dessert: Banana Rice Cream
- Beverage: Herbal Rice Tea

Day 6

- Breakfast: Peachy Rice Breakfast Bowl
- Lunch: Asian Rice and Cabbage Salad
- Dinner: Rice and Chickpea Stuffed Avocados
- Snacks: Mediterranean Rice Tabbouleh
- Dessert: Rice and Lentil Salad
- Beverage: Cold Rice and Pea Soup

Day 7

- Breakfast: Savory Rice and Spinach Pancakes
- Lunch: Mediterranean Rice Tabbouleh
- Dinner: Cold Rice and Pea Soup
- Snacks: Asian Rice and Cabbage Salad

- Dessert: Fruit and Rice Pudding

- Beverage: Rice Milk Smoothie

Day 8

- Breakfast: Rice and Nutmeg Porridge

- Lunch: Cold Rice and Pea Soup

- Dinner: Lentil and Rice Stew

- Snacks: Sweet Potato Rice Cakes

- Dessert: Baked Apples with Rice and Cinnamon

- Beverage: Golden Rice Tea

Day 9

- Breakfast: Rice and Berry Parfait

- Lunch: Rice and Lentil Salad

- Dinner: Tomato Basil Rice

- Snacks: Baked Rice Chips

- Dessert: Rice and Carrot Halwa

- Beverage: Rice Water with Lemon and Mint

Day 10

- Breakfast: Tropical Rice Pudding

- Lunch: Vegetable Stir-Fry over Brown Rice

- Dinner: Spinach and Lemon Rice

- Snacks: Rice and Zucchini Fritters

- Dessert: Banana Rice Cream

- Beverage: Cucumber Rice Water

Day 11

- Breakfast: Peachy Rice Breakfast Bowl

- Lunch: Mushroom Rice Soup

- Dinner: Rice Primavera
- Snacks: Rice and Kale Chips
- Dessert: Rice Flour Pancakes
- Beverage: Herbal Rice Tea

Day 12

- Breakfast: Savory Rice and Spinach Pancakes
- Lunch: Curried Rice Salad
- Dinner: Cauliflower Rice Stir-Fry
- Snacks: Mediterranean Rice Tabbouleh
- Dessert: Fruit and Rice Pudding
- Beverage: Rice Milk Smoothie

Day 13

- Breakfast: Rice Cakes with Avocado
- Lunch: Asian Rice and Cabbage Salad
- Dinner: Rice and Chickpea Stuffed Avocados
- Snacks: Cucumber Rice Vinegar Salad
- Dessert: Rice and Lentil Salad
- Beverage: Cold Rice and Pea Soup

Day 14

- Breakfast: Apple Cinnamon Rice Breakfast
- Lunch: Rice-Stuffed Bell Peppers
- Dinner: Lentil and Rice Stew
- Snacks: Sweet Potato Rice Cakes
- Dessert: Rice Flour Pancakes
- Beverage: Golden Rice Tea

Day 15

- Breakfast: Tropical Rice Smoothie
- Lunch: Mediterranean Rice Tabbouleh
- Dinner: Tomato Basil Rice
- Snacks: Rice and Kale Chips
- Dessert: Baked Apples with Rice and Cinnamon
- Beverage: Rice Water with Lemon and Mint (refreshing and hydrating)

Day 16

- Breakfast: Savory Rice and Spinach Pancakes
- Lunch: Cold Rice and Pea Soup
- Dinner: Cauliflower Rice Stir-Fry
- Snacks: Cucumber Rice Vinegar Salad
- Dessert: Banana Rice Cream
- Beverage: Herbal Rice Tea

Day 17

- Breakfast: Rice and Berry Parfait
- Lunch: Rice and Lentil Salad
- Dinner: Spinach and Lemon Rice
- Snacks: Baked Rice Chips
- Dessert: Rice and Carrot Halwa
- Beverage: Cucumber Rice Water

Day 18

- Breakfast: Rice Cakes with Avocado
- Lunch: Vegetable Stir-Fry over Brown Rice
- Dinner: Lentil and Rice Stew

- Snacks: Sweet Potato Rice Cakes

- Dessert: Rice Flour Pancakes

- Beverage: Golden Rice Tea

Day 19

- Breakfast: Peachy Rice Breakfast Bowl

- Lunch: Curried Rice Salad

- Dinner: Rice Primavera

- Snacks: Mediterranean Rice Tabbouleh

- Dessert: Fruit and Rice Pudding

- Beverage: Rice Milk Smoothie

Day 20

- Breakfast: Basic Brown Rice Porridge

- Lunch: Mushroom Rice Soup

- Dinner: Rice and Chickpea Stuffed Avocados

- Snacks: Asian Rice and Cabbage Salad

- Dessert: Baked Apples with Rice and Cinnamon

- Beverage: Rice Water with Lemon and Mint

Day 21

- Breakfast: Apple Cinnamon Rice Breakfast

- Lunch: Asian Rice and Cabbage Salad

- Dinner: Cold Rice and Pea Soup

- Snacks: Rice and Zucchini Fritters

- Dessert: Banana Rice Cream

- Beverage: Herbal Rice Tea

FREQUENTLY ASKED QUESTIONS (FAQs)

Addressing Common Concerns and Misconceptions

1. Isn't eating too much rice bad for you? Eating a variety of foods is key to a balanced diet, but rice, especially whole grain rice like brown rice, can be a healthy part of your diet. The rice diet focuses on portion control, variety (including other grains, fruits, and vegetables), and limiting processed foods, which helps mitigate the risks associated with consuming too much of any single food.

2. Will I get enough protein on the rice diet? Yes, the rice diet can provide adequate protein if carefully planned. While rice itself contains protein, the diet also includes beans, lentils, and other plant-based protein sources to ensure you meet your protein needs.

3. Can the rice diet lead to nutrient deficiencies? Any restrictive diet can lead to nutrient deficiencies if not properly planned. The rice diet encourages the inclusion of a wide range of fruits, vegetables, and legumes to ensure you receive a broad spectrum of vitamins, minerals, and other nutrients. It's always a good idea to consult with a healthcare provider or a dietitian when making significant dietary changes.

4. Is the rice diet considered a fad diet? The rice diet has been around since the 1930s and was initially developed for medical purposes, specifically for hypertension and kidney disease management. While it has seen variations and gained popularity for weight loss, its core principles of whole foods, plant-based eating, and limiting processed foods align with general healthy eating guidelines.

5. How does the rice diet compare to low-carb or keto diets? The rice diet is significantly higher in carbohydrates and lower in fats than low-carb or keto diets. It emphasizes whole, plant-based foods and minimizes animal products and fats. The choice between these diets should be based on individual health goals, nutritional needs, and personal preference, ideally under the guidance of a healthcare professional.

6. Will I feel hungry all the time on the rice diet? The rice diet focuses on high-fiber, whole foods that are meant to be filling and satisfying. Including a variety of whole grains, vegetables, and legumes can help keep you feeling full throughout the day. Drinking plenty of water and eating regular meals can also help manage hunger.

7. Can I follow the rice diet if I have diabetes? The rice diet, particularly when focusing on whole grains and fiber-rich foods, can be adapted for individuals with diabetes. It's important to monitor blood sugar levels and possibly adjust medication dosages accordingly. Consulting with a healthcare provider is essential when following any diet with diabetes.

8. How quickly will I lose weight on the rice diet? Weight loss can vary based on individual factors like metabolism, starting weight, and adherence to the diet. Initially, you may see rapid weight loss, much of which is water weight. Sustainable, healthy weight loss is typically around 1-2 pounds per week.

9. Can I exercise while on the rice diet? Yes, exercise is encouraged as part of a healthy lifestyle. However, since the rice diet is low in calories, particularly in its initial phases, you may need to adjust the intensity and duration of your workouts. Listen to your body and consult with a healthcare provider to determine the best exercise plan for you.

10. Do I need to be on the rice diet forever to maintain my weight loss? The rice diet's initial phases are more restrictive and are not intended to be followed long-term. The maintenance phase is designed to be a sustainable, healthy eating plan that can be followed indefinitely. Learning healthy eating habits and making lifestyle changes during the diet can help you maintain your weight loss over time.

Addressing these questions can help individuals feel more informed and confident about whether the rice diet is a suitable choice for their health goals and lifestyle.

CONCLUSIONS

The Future of the Rice Diet

Looking ahead, the Rice Diet's principles seem more relevant than ever in a world grappling with rising rates of chronic diseases linked to poor dietary habits. Its emphasis on whole grains, fruits, vegetables, and legumes not only aligns with global dietary guidelines aimed at promoting health and preventing disease but also with growing environmental concerns advocating for more sustainable eating practices.

Integrating the lessons from the Rice Diet into our daily lives offers a blueprint for nurturing our bodies, respecting the planet, and fostering a healthier relationship with food. It's about recognizing that each meal is an opportunity to fuel our bodies with nutrient-rich foods, to enjoy the flavors and textures that nature provides, and to honor the role that diet plays in our overall well-being.

Adopting the Rice Diet's principles doesn't require a radical overhaul of your eating habits overnight. It's a journey that begins with small, manageable steps: choosing brown rice over white, incorporating more fruits and vegetables into your meals, reducing the intake of processed foods, and being mindful of portion sizes. It's about making conscious choices that align with your health goals and ethical values.

For many, the biggest hurdle is breaking free from the cycle of quick fixes and fad diets, which promise rapid results but seldom deliver lasting change. The Rice Diet teaches us the value of patience and consistency. It reminds us that meaningful transformation takes time and that health is not just a destination but a continuous journey.

As you embark on this journey, remember that setbacks are part of the process. There will be days when convenience wins over nutrition, and that's okay. What matters is your commitment to getting back on track, to learning from each experience, and to moving forward with a clearer understanding of what works best for your body.

If you're considering integrating the Rice Diet's lessons into your life, or if you're already on this path, know that you are not alone. There are countless others on similar journeys, each with their own challenges and triumphs. Seek out communities, whether online or in-person, where you can share experiences, exchange recipes, and offer support to one another. Remember, the journey to health is always richer and more enjoyable when shared.

To anyone standing at the crossroads, contemplating the step towards a healthier lifestyle through the Rice Diet or any other nutritional plan, know that your aspirations for better health are valid and achievable. Change, though daunting, is possible with determination, patience, and the right support.

Let the principles of the Rice Diet serve not just as dietary guidelines but as a metaphor for life: nourish yourself with what truly benefits you, discard what doesn't serve your well-being, and recognize that every small choice can contribute to a larger change.

As you move forward, let this quote inspire you: *"The food you eat can be either the safest and most powerful form of medicine or the slowest form of poison."* – Ann Wigmore. Let this wisdom guide your choices, reminding you of the profound impact your diet has on your health and life.

Remember, the journey towards health and wellness is a marathon, not a sprint. Embrace the lessons from the Rice Diet with an open heart and mind, and let them guide you towards a future where food is not just sustenance but a source of vitality, joy, and well-being.

Weekly Meal Planner

Grocery List

	Breakfast	Lunch	Dinner	Snacks
mon				
tue				
wed				
thu				
fri				
sat				
sun				

Weekly Meal Planner

Grocery List

Breakfast	Lunch	Dinner	Snacks
mon			
tue			
wed			
thu			
fri			
sat			
sun			

Weekly Meal Planner

Grocery List

	Breakfast	Lunch	Dinner	Snacks
mon				
tue				
wed				
thu				
fri				
sat				
sun				

Weekly Meal Planner

Grocery List

	Breakfast	Lunch	Dinner	Snacks
mon				
tue				
wed				
thu				
fri				
sat				
sun				

Weekly Meal Planner

Grocery List

	Breakfast	Lunch	Dinner	Snacks
mon				
tue				
wed				
thu				
fri				
sat				
sun				

Weekly Meal Planner

Grocery List

	Breakfast	Lunch	Dinner	Snacks
mon				
tue				
wed				
thu				
fri				
sat				
sun				

Weekly Meal Planner

Grocery List

	Breakfast	Lunch	Dinner	Snacks
mon				
tue				
wed				
thu				
fri				
sat				
sun				

Weekly Meal Planner

Grocery List

	Breakfast	Lunch	Dinner	Snacks
mon				
tue				
wed				
thu				
fri				
sat				
sun				

Weekly Meal Planner

Grocery List

		Breakfast	Lunch	Dinner	Snacks
mon					
tue					
wed					
thu					
fri					
sat					
sun					

Weekly Meal Planner

Grocery List

	Breakfast	Lunch	Dinner	Snacks
mon				
tue				
wed				
thu				
fri				
sat				
sun				